# Mig[illegible]s



## A self-help guide to feeling better

Wendy Green

Foreword by Professor Anne MacGregor, specialist in headache and women's health, and honorary professor at the Centre for Neuroscience and Trauma

PERSONAL HEALTH GUIDES

MIGRAINES: A SELF-HELP GUIDE TO FEELING BETTER

First published in 2009 as *50 Things You Can Do Today to Manage Migraines*


Vie Books is an imprint of Summersdale Publishers Ltd

Summersdale Publishers Ltd
46 West Street
Chichester
West Sussex
PO19 1RP
UK

www.summersdale.com

Printed and bound by CPI Group (UK) Ltd, Croydon, CR0 4YY

ISBN: 978-1-84953-808-4



Disclaimer
Every effort has been made to ensure that the information in this book is accurate and current at the time of publication. The author and the publisher cannot accept responsibility for any misuse or misunderstanding of any information contained herein, or any loss, damage or injury, be it health, financial or otherwise, suffered by any individual or group acting upon or relying on information contained herein. None of the opinions or suggestions in this book is intended to replace medical opinion. If you have concerns about your health, please seek professional advice.

*To my husband Gordon – thanks for being so supportive*

# Acknowledgements

I would like to thank Professor Anne MacGregor, specialist in headache and women's health and honorary professor at the Centre for Neuroscience and Trauma at the Blizard Institute of Cell and Molecular Science, Barts and the London School of Medicine and Dentistry, for her expert advice and help – especially with regard to medical treatments for migraine. I'd also like to thank Jennifer Barclay for commissioning the original book and Claire Plimmer for commissioning this edition. I'm also grateful to Lucy York, Anna Martin, Laura Booth, Debbie Chapman and Jennifer Jahn for their very helpful editorial input.

# Contents

# Author's Note

I have suffered from migraines since the age of 15. At the start of my first attack, my field of vision must have been affected because I could only see half of everything I looked at. It was a terrifying experience. I initially thought I was somehow going blind until, of course, the aura faded away, to be replaced by a pulsating, one-sided headache. My next migraine did not happen until I was 22 and pregnant; again my field of vision was halved. Over the next 20 years I experienced only a few migraines – but they were severe and left me incapacitated for days. During the menopause, my migraines increased first to one a month and then gradually they became a weekly event. My GP prescribed triptans, which worked once an attack was under way, but I still felt the effects for a few days afterwards, so I was keen to prevent them from happening in the first place.

I gradually realised that missing meals was a trigger, as was feeling stressed. I started making sure I never went too long without food and learned to recognise when I was feeling stressed and how to deal with it. I also began taking a supplement called 5HTP. Fairly quickly my attacks became less frequent.

Unfortunately, in 2013, my migraine frequency increased dramatically – to as many as three a week. I tried numerous supplements, dietary changes, stress-management techniques and even visited a chiropractor, but nothing helped. In desperation

I asked my GP if I could be referred for acupuncture. After receiving the four treatments covered by the NHS, I noticed that my migraines were both less frequent and less severe. However, once the treatment ended, they quickly worsened again, so I decided to pay privately for traditional Chinese acupuncture. Initially my migraines became more frequent and intense before improving dramatically. I found that having acupuncture every three weeks reduced the number of attacks to around three a month – a huge improvement, but I still wanted to try to reduce them further; two months ago I also began taking 3 mg of melatonin every night before bed and have experienced just one migraine since. I am now hopeful that I have finally got my migraines under control without having to take the preventative anti-epileptic drug with worrying possible side effects, that I was prescribed by my consultant.

Migraine is an individual condition, and what works for one person may not work for another. In this book I provide an overview of the condition and present a wide variety of tips and advice, including dietary information and techniques from complementary therapies, to help fellow sufferers gain better control of their symptoms.

Throughout this book I refer to the condition as 'migraines'; however, in medical literature it is often described in the singular, i.e. 'migraine'.

Wendy Green

# Foreword

Migraines affect different people in different ways. Some people find that no matter what they do to treat attacks, they are laid up for a day or so and unable to function normally; others can take a couple of painkillers and get on with their day. But no matter how mild or severe the attacks are or whether they seek medical advice, most people who suffer from migraines rely heavily on self-help strategies.

Using her own experience to draw upon, Wendy Green outlines the variety of treatments that are available over the counter, and also gives an overview of what is available from a GP. Research shows that sufferers are often satisfied with drugs that don't provide a great deal of benefit. Hence, it is important to explore the wealth of strategies that are available in order to ensure that you are receiving the optimum treatment.

It may not yet be possible to 'cure' migraines, but it is possible to lead a normal life despite them.

Professor Anne MacGregor,
specialist in headache and women's health, and
honorary professor at the Centre for Neuroscience and Trauma

# Introduction

Research suggests that, in the UK, around one in five women, one in twelve men and one in nine children suffer from migraines. Sufferers are most likely to experience their first attack during their childhood or teenage years. Roughly equal numbers of boys and girls experience migraines until puberty, when it becomes more common in girls. Overall, around six million people – 10 per cent of the population – are thought to suffer from the condition. On average, sufferers experience 13 attacks a year, yet some can go for several years without a migraine.

A study in 2007 reported that less than 50 per cent of people with migraine symptoms seek medical help. This is likely to be for various reasons. For example, some individuals may only have a few migraines in their lifetime, and do so without even realising it. Also, migraine can be inherited; 50–60 per cent of migraineurs have a parent and 80 per cent have a sibling who also has the condition. Many such sufferers do not consult their GP because they believe little can be done and they tend to suffer in silence. Even when some sufferers do eventually visit their GP, their condition may be misdiagnosed as a tension or cluster headache.

**Famous migraine sufferers**

In 2015, when *Britain's Got Talent* contestant Danny Posthill said that he'd been bedridden with a migraine attack until 3 p.m. on the day of the final, music and TV producer Simon Cowell, a judge on the show, revealed that he'd also been laid up all day with a migraine.

In May 2006, Hollywood actor and director Ben Affleck made the headlines not for his acting talents but because he was rushed into hospital after complaining of pains in his head. It was revealed later the same day that he had received treatment for a migraine.

He later described how the making of the film *Gone Baby Gone* – his directing debut – had triggered the attack, saying, 'I put a lot of pressure on myself. I overplanned, I gave myself migraines and generally caused myself a lot of physical pain.'

Lewis Carroll, the renowned author of *Alice's Adventures in Wonderland*, was known to suffer from migraines. It has even been suggested that some of Alice's experiences – such as growing very big and then becoming very small – were inspired by Carroll's migraine symptoms. Alice in Wonderland Syndrome is now a neurological term used to describe a distorted perception of reality, like that experienced by sufferers during a migraine aura.

Julius Caesar, Princess Margaret, Elvis Presley, Elizabeth Taylor, Elle Macpherson and *Friends* actress Lisa Kudrow are just a few other well-known migraineurs.

## Chapter 1

# About Migraines

A migraine is a complex, episodic (intermittent), neurological condition characterised by an intensely painful, throbbing, one-sided headache. However, migraine isn't just a headache – it is a collection of symptoms and the headache isn't always the predominant feature. Other symptoms can include nausea and vomiting; visual disturbance; pins and needles down one side of the body; increased sensitivity to sound, light and smells; a stiff and aching neck; drooping eyelids; lethargy and exhaustion.

## Do migraines cause permanent damage?

Migraines can be debilitating and terrifying, but there is no evidence that they cause any permanent damage to the body. Common fears are loss of sight, or that they are indicating the onset of a stroke or the presence of a brain tumour. However, these are rarely linked to migraine and most sufferers return to their normal selves in between attacks. The two main types of migraine are:

**Migraine with aura** – otherwise known as a 'classical migraine' and, incorrectly, as a focal migraine; the term 'focal' is also used to describe the neurological symptoms of a stroke, whereas 'aura' relates only to those specific to migraines.

**Migraine without aura** – also known as a 'common migraine'.

Other forms of migraine include:

**Menstrual migraine** – migraines that occur between two days before and three days after the start of the menstrual period.

**Menstrually-related migraine** – these migraines develop at the time of a period and other times during the menstrual cycle and are clearly linked to hormonal fluctuations. For more in-depth information, see Chapter 5 – Migraine and Hormones.

**Basilar-type migraine** – this form of the condition can involve speech problems, double vision, dizziness and even fainting. It is rare, with only around one in 400 migraineurs suffering from it. It is thought to be caused when the basilar artery – a blood vessel at the base of the brain – goes into spasm, leading to a reduced blood supply to the brain.

**Hemiplegic migraine** – is a very rare form of the condition, often genetic, where the migraineur experiences weakness down one side of the body that may last for several days. Other symptoms include double vision or blindness, impaired hearing and mobility and numbness around the mouth, causing problems with speaking or swallowing.

**Retinal migraine** – is also uncommon though some studies suggest that may be partly because it is not always correctly diagnosed. Retinal migraines (as with all migraines) affect more women than men and it seems to be more common in women who have had migraines with auras. In retinal migraines, visual problems develop before the headache part of the attack and there may be total but temporary blindness, often in one eye. There may also be temporary blind spots. It is thought the visual problems are due to the muscles around the eye contracting and disrupting blood flow. A retinal migraine may differ from a migraine with aura in that the visual disturbance tends to affect just one eye rather than both. Exercise, or any other form of physical exertion, may prompt a retinal migraine.

**Ocular (opthalmoplegic) migraine** – is another rare type of migraine. It usually occurs in children aged from six to twelve years, but can also occur in adults. The pain is often around the eye and may be accompanied by weakness in one of the eye muscles, as well as double vision, nausea and vomiting.

## The stages of a migraine

There are five distinct stages that can happen during a classical migraine attack. These are the prodromal, aura, headache, resolution and recovery phases. There is no aura in a common migraine.

## 1. Prodromal (premonitory) symptoms

These can start up to 24 hours before an attack. Some people find they are bursting with energy and rush around doing far more than usual. Others may find themselves sinking into a low mood and feeling tired or craving food – especially sweet things. Irritability and general aches and pains, particularly in the neck, are also common features.

**Neck Pain**

Neck pain is fairly common among migraineurs and can be both a migraine trigger and a symptom of the migraine itself, occurring before, during or after an attack. The pain can be felt in the muscles, discs, bones or nerves in the neck. In my case, I often experience tightness in the neck muscles on one side, which sometimes develops into pain that travels down my arm. At other times the pain radiates from between my shoulder blades right up to my neck and head and then across my forehead. Poor posture or arthritis is just one of the causes of neck pain that can trigger migraines.

In a 2010 study of 113 migraine patients, published in *Headache: The Journal of Head and Face Pain*, 75 per cent experienced neck pain before or during attacks. Some participants said their neck felt tight, while others experienced stiffness.

Note: A stiff neck can signify a more serious or potentially life-threatening condition. If you experience a stiff neck with a fever and headache, seek immediate medical attention.

## 2. Aura

Aura is the term used to describe sensory changes experienced by about one in ten migraineurs prior to the onset of the headache itself. Common aura symptoms include:

**Visual disturbance** – this is the most common type of aura symptom and can include blind spots, silvery flashing lights, zigzag patterns or even tunnel vision. This symptom can be quite alarming – especially when you experience it for the first time.

**Pins and needles or numbness down one side** – this often follows visual disturbance and usually begins in the hand, travelling up the arm and, in some cases, reaching the face, lips and tongue. Sometimes the numbness travels down the leg. This symptom can also occur with hemiplegic migraine.

**Speech disturbance (dysphasia)** – the sufferer has difficulty in finding the right words; this is the third most common aura symptom.

**Confusion and clumsiness** – this may also be experienced by some sufferers.

All of these symptoms indicate that the brain isn't functioning normally. If any of these symptoms continue for longer than an hour, see your GP, as they may indicate something more serious.

**Note**

Most people who suffer from migraine with aura also have attacks without auras. This is an important point to bear in mind; I did not realise this was the case at first and had always only taken my migraine medication after the start of any visual disturbance. On a couple of occasions I had a severe one-sided pulsing headache and didn't take medication soon enough because I didn't realise I was having a migraine. As a result, the attack lasted longer. In one sense the aura is useful as it forewarns that a migraine is imminent.

## 3. Headache

The headache is usually only experienced on one side of the head, though some people experience pain on both sides. The pain is usually intense and extends across the forehead or temples. It can last between four and 72 hours, but this can be shortened considerably by taking painkillers or using alternative treatments – such as the application of one or two drops of peppermint or lavender oil to the site of the pain – as early on as possible. See Chapter 6 – Medical and Other Treatments and Chapter 7 – DIY Complementary Therapies.

The headache is also accompanied by at least one of these other symptoms:

**Stomach upset** – including nausea, vomiting and diarrhoea. Nausea accompanies the headache in around 95 per cent of migraineurs. There may also be a heightened sense of smell (osmophobia) that is possibly linked to the nausea – some people find they are aware of smells that they would not normally notice. About a quarter of sufferers vomit and around one in five have diarrhoea. Some find eating a little plain food – digestive biscuits or dry toast – helps, while others are unable to face food. Chewing raw ginger root or eating ginger biscuits may also ease the nausea, see Chapter 2 – The Food Factor for more information.

The nausea is linked to the digestive system slowing down during an attack. This also makes the absorption of food or medication more difficult.

**Photophobia** – increased sensitivity to light – is common in about 80 per cent of migraineurs. Many sufferers find themselves instinctively wanting to escape a light environment. Looking at a computer screen or watching TV may be uncomfortable.

**Phonophobia** – increased sensitivity to noise – seems to be part of the heightening of senses that many people experience and that causes sufferers to seek out a quiet and dark place to rest during a migraine. Go to bed, if you can, and draw the bedroom curtains.

**Droopy or puffy eyelids** – the eyelids can appear swollen and droopy or just feel heavy.

## 4. Resolution

The way an attack comes to an end varies from one person to another. Some people feel better after taking painkillers, others only feel better after lying down in a darkened room or being sick.

## 5. The recovery phase (postdrome)

Once the headache has gone, it can take a few days to return to normal. During this time you will probably feel washed out and lethargic – some people describe it as a migraine hangover, though some sufferers report feeling more energetic immediately after an attack. Other postdrome symptoms include sore muscles, scalp tenderness, mood changes and general malaise. As you return to normal, treat yourself kindly and don't overdo things.

## Episodic and Chronic Migraine

Migraines are further defined by how often the sufferer experiences them.

Episodic migraine is defined as fewer than 15 headache days per month. Chronic migraine is categorised as more than 15 headache days per month over a period of three months, of which more than eight are migrainous (in the absence of medication overuse).

Although chronic migraine, also known as transformed migraine, is thought to affect less than one per cent of the population, this still equates to more than 610,000 chronic migraine sufferers in the UK. The severity and frequency of the symptoms of chronic migraines mean they can be very disabling.

Chronic migraineurs are more likely to be absent from work and school and experience disruption of their leisure and social activities than episodic migraine sufferers. The after effects of chronic migraine are also thought to halve the productivity of sufferers at work or school. For some sufferers, being unable to function normally for more than half of the month means they are unable to work at all, so they have to rely on disability living allowance. In recognition of the serious impact chronic migraine can have on sufferers' lives, the World Health Organisation (WHO) has categorised it as more disabling than blindness, paraplegia, angina or rheumatoid arthritis.

Each year, there are around 2.5 to 4.6 per cent of people with episodic migraines whose condition progresses to chronic migraines, while a similar percentage reverts back to episodic migraines. There are many individual factors that could be involved in why migraines become chronic; some large-scale studies have identified links with chronic overuse of acute medication (i.e. painkillers/triptans), chronic sleep problems, obesity, anxiety/depression, and hypothyroidism. There is also evidence that a progressive increase in migraine frequency could be linked to the fact that the brain 'learns pain'. However, it has also been shown that early therapeutic intervention – before migraine attacks have reached a critical level of frequency – may help to prevent them becoming chronic.

## Migraines in children and teenagers

These differ from migraines in adults; children may experience vomiting or abdominal pain without a headache, or they may suffer from a headache that affects the whole head instead of being one sided. Attacks in children and teenagers can be considerably shorter than those in adults – some last for less than an hour.

The advice for dealing with migraines in children is the same as for adults: identify and avoid the triggers and select suitable treatments. There is advice on how to do this throughout the book.

The main triggers in children are likely to be eating insufficient food, not drinking enough fluids and, occasionally, a food sensitivity (see Chapter 2 – The Food Factor). Stress linked to worrying about exams could also be a factor (see Chapter 4 – Mind Over Migraine). In teenage girls it could be linked to menstruation (see Chapter 5 – Migraine and Hormones).

The tips outlined in this book, such as lying down in a darkened room and taking painkillers early on, also apply to child migraineurs. It is best to stick to basic medications for young children suffering from a migraine, like soluble paracetamol, perhaps 'disguised' in a fizzy drink. Ibuprofen is also safe, but aspirin should not be taken by children under 16 years of age because of the risk of developing Reye's Syndrome. Other drugs – like triptans – are generally not recommended for children under the age of 18, except for sumatriptan nasal spray.

**Note**

Always consult a GP if a child in your care has recurring headaches or you are unsure of the diagnosis. The Migraine Action Association runs a website for children who suffer from migraines called Migraine 4 Kids. Further details can be found in the Directory at the end of the book.

## What causes migraines?

No one knows exactly why migraines happen, but several theories have been put forward involving genetics, blood vessels in the brain, the nervous system, a brain chemical called serotonin – also known as 5-hydroxytryptamine (5HT) – and a heart defect.

### Genetics

It seems that many migraine sufferers inherit a predisposition to the condition as it often runs in families.

### The blood vessels

There is a long-held view that migraines occur when the blood vessels in the brain first narrow (constrict) and then expand (swell). This leads to fluctuations in blood flow to the brain, which result in migraine symptoms.

### The nervous system

This view actually backs up the blood vessel theory by suggesting how changes in the blood vessels come about. It is thought that the chain of events leading to an attack begins with oversensitive brain cells triggering nerves to release brain chemicals. These chemicals cause the blood vessels in the head to swell, leading to pain, throbbing and other migraine symptoms. The hypothalamus is part of the brain that is linked to much of the nervous system and it controls, among other things, appetite and emotions. This may explain prodromal symptoms, such as food cravings and mood changes.

### Serotonin

It has been suggested that levels of a brain chemical called serotonin, or 5-hydroxytryptamine (5HT), are low at the beginning of an attack. Serotonin is important for normal brain function and affects the size of the blood vessels. It is thought that drugs called triptans – also known as 5HT agonists – constrict the blood vessels in the brain by balancing the levels of serotonin. An injection of serotonin has been shown to end an attack, but it is not used as a treatment as it has a number of adverse side effects. For more information about serotonin and how you can safely increase your intake, see Chapter 2 – The Food Factor and Chapter 3 – Supplementary Benefits.

### A heart defect

Research has suggested a possible link between migraine with aura and a hole in the heart, which is known medically as a patent foramen ovale (PFO). PFO is a small hole in the wall that divides the two upper chambers of the heart (the atria). All babies have this hole whilst in the womb, so that blood is circulated more efficiently. The hole usually closes after birth, but in some people it stays open. Tests show that 60 per cent of migraine sufferers have larger than average PFOs, which is six times as many as the general population. It is thought that the problem can lead to impurities not being filtered out of the blood properly. In those without a PFO, all of the blood returning to the heart after being pumped around the body is cleaned and filtered by the lungs to remove small clots and other debris. However, in those with the condition, unfiltered blood may get through the hole. It is believed that when this unfiltered blood reaches the brain it can trigger a migraine in some people. It is possible to close a PFO using corrective surgery but, following a trial involving 147 people with severe migraines, concerns have been raised over the risks involved, especially given the small reduction in migraine frequency that was reported (see Chapter 7 – Medical and Other Treatments).

It is possible that all of these factors could be interrelated. For example, a migraine sufferer could inherit an oversensitivity to stimuli, such as bright light, loud noise or physiological disturbances, including blood sugar changes, altered sleep patterns or dehydration. Any of these could trigger the release of serotonin – causing the blood vessels first to narrow and then widen – which then leads to a migraine. In some cases a migraineur could inherit a PFO, which could lead to similar changes in the brain and trigger an attack.

# 1 Determine whether it is a migraine

## DIY Migraine Test

This is based on a 'self-administered screener' for migraines, which was developed by scientists in 2003. If you answer 'yes' to at least two of the following three questions, it is likely your headache was a migraine.

1. Did you feel nauseous?

2. Did light bother you more than usual?

3. Did your headache limit your ability to do what you wanted for at least one day?

## What else could it be?

There are other types of severe headache, including tension and cluster headaches, which could be mistaken for a migraine.

### Tension headache

With tension headaches, the sufferer experiences a dull and heavy pain and a feeling of pressure – as if a band is being tightened around their head. The pain tends to worsen as the day goes on and can last for several days. There may also be a dislike of light and noise, but not to the same degree as with a migraine. The pain is also likely to be less severe and is not usually one sided. However, a tension headache may sometimes be misdiagnosed as a migraine without aura. The cause, as the name suggests, is usually stress and tension, and painkillers may not help. The pain tends to arise from the neck muscles going into spasm. As well as stress, poor posture and neck injuries are common causes of muscular tension in the neck. Improving posture and finding ways to relax and manage stress may help both to prevent and relieve the pain.

**Cluster headache**

These headaches, as the name suggests, tend to occur in clusters, i.e. several attacks over one or two months and then none at all. They are more common in men than women, but are relatively rare, with less than one per cent of the population experiencing them. The pain is one sided and throbbing and centred around the eye, but it can spread to the temple or jaw. The pain can be very severe, the eye can redden and water and the eyelid may droop. The nose may be blocked or running and the face may flush or sweat. As with a migraine, the pain of a cluster headache can be excruciating, but it is not accompanied by the other symptoms that characterise a migraine attack. Over-the-counter painkillers are unlikely to help, but prescribed medications called triptans – also used to treat migraines – can be effective. The contact details for OUCH, The Organisation for the Understanding of Cluster Headaches, can be found in the Directory at the end of the book.

## ❷ Identify your triggers

Here is a summary of common migraine triggers:

**Not enough food** – missing meals and snacking, especially on sugary foods instead of eating proper meals, can lead to a drop in blood sugar, which can precipitate an attack. It is recommended that migraine sufferers eat regularly: at least every four hours during the day and to go no longer than 12 hours without food overnight. See Chapter 2 – The Food Factor, for more information on how your eating habits can be implicated in migraines.

**Certain foods** – some people believe that foods containing an amino acid called tyramine (aged cheese, processed meats, etc.) can trigger an attack. Others claim that an allergic reaction to particular foods can lead to a migraine. Food additives may also be a factor for some people. More information about tyramine, food allergies and food additives can be found in Chapter 2 – The Food Factor.

**Some alcoholic drinks** – red wine, beer, stout and ale also contain tyramine and may therefore be a trigger in some susceptible people. See Chapter 2 – The Food Factor to find out more.

**Smoking** – and second-hand smoke from cigarettes can trigger a migraine in some people. Nicotine, a constituent of tobacco, is thought to cause the narrowing of blood vessels in the brain.

**Dehydration** – not drinking enough fluids can be a factor in some people's migraine attacks. It is recommended that people drink at least 1.5 litres of water a day. This can include tea and coffee. Although both have been linked to dehydration because of the diuretic effect of the caffeine they contain, research suggests that three or four cups a day should not cause a problem. However, some people find coffee can precipitate a migraine (see Chapter 2 – The Food Factor). Alcohol is also a diuretic. To avoid dehydration, drink moderate amounts of caffeinated drinks and plenty of water (see point 38: Cope with summer, Christmas and the working day, in Chapter 6 – Tackling Other Triggers).

**Emotional stress** – migraine often develops after, rather than during, a period of stress. This is probably why some people suffer at weekends or whilst on holiday. A survey by the Migraine Action Association backs this up with 37 out of 39 migraine sufferers saying they'd had an attack whilst on holiday. Anger, worry, tension, excitement, shock and depression can all play a part in triggering migraines. To find out more see Chapter 4 – Mind Over Migraine.

**Strenuous exercise** – regular exercise is thought to help lower the risk of attacks, but doing an exceptional amount of exercise can be a trigger.

**A change in sleep pattern** – going to bed later, or getting up earlier than usual, can lead to an attack, as can having a lie-in. Research in Belgrade, Serbia, suggested that migraineurs who sleep for longer than nine hours have more migraine attacks than those who sleep less. Jet lag or shift work can also have the same effect.

**Neck and shoulder pain** – muscular tension in the neck and shoulders can be a factor. Neck pain is especially common among office workers who sit for hours at a computer. It is also common among drivers. Chiropractors suggest that tense neck and shoulder muscles can lead to constricted blood vessels in the head, which may then trigger a migraine. See Chapter 6 – Tackling Other Triggers.

**Dental problems** – changes to an individual's bite can cause muscular tension in the head and lead to a migraine. Grinding your teeth during sleep can cause tension in the cheek muscles, which could also set off an attack. Problems with wisdom teeth may be a trigger for some. Your dentist may be able to help resolve these problems.

**Bright lights** – some people appear to be sensitive to bright lights, especially harsh strip lights and flickering lights or light emitted from a computer screen. Most migraineurs become sensitive to light during an attack. See also Chapter 6 – Tackling Other Triggers.

**Changes in the weather and extremes of temperature** – very hot or cold conditions or strong winds, as well as sudden changes in temperature, humidity and atmospheric pressure, all seem to be triggers for some people. See also Chapter 6 – Tackling Other Triggers.

**Strong smells/fumes** – responses to a survey by the manufacturers of Migraleve, an over-the-counter medication for the relief of migraines, revealed that perfume, aftershave, cigarette smoke, aerosol sprays, household products and petrol are fairly common migraine triggers. See also Chapter 6 – Tackling Other Triggers.

**Loud noise** – for example loud music.

**Hormonal changes** – some women find their attacks become more frequent when taking the contraceptive pill or HRT. In such cases the general advice is to stop taking it. Women who have migraines with auras are advised not to take the pill and to adopt alternative contraception methods. Hormonal changes due to menstruation, pregnancy and the menopause can also be implicated.

Some women suffer from attacks just before a period, when their oestrogen levels drop. Some women find their symptoms improve during pregnancy, whilst others find they worsen. The menopause is another time when some women find they experience more attacks, again this is a time when oestrogen levels fluctuate or drop. For more information see Chapter 5 – Migraines and Hormones.

**Medications** – such as hormone replacement therapy (HRT), some sleeping tablets and the contraceptive pill. If you think you are affected, speak to your GP as they should be able to prescribe alternative medication.

Identifying your own particular triggers can be difficult, especially when it often seems that the same triggers don't always lead to an attack. Dr MacGregor suggests that sufferers have a migraine threshold, which is raised or lowered by various internal and external factors, or even some medications. Usually, more than one trigger has to occur before a person is pushed over their individual threshold and develops a migraine. For example, your triggers could be lack of sleep, stress and not eating enough. Each of these factors individually might not lead to a migraine. But if you sleep badly one night, then have a busy and stressful day at work, and as a result don't eat enough, you may suffer a migraine, depending on your current threshold level. It is even possible that everyone could potentially suffer from migraines, but most people have a very high threshold where a lot of triggers would need to be present at one time, so they rarely, if ever, experience an attack. Following a healthy lifestyle and managing stress successfully may raise your threshold and therefore reduce the number of attacks.

## 3 Keep a migraine trigger diary

One way of discovering your particular triggers is to keep a migraine trigger diary for some time, depending on the frequency of your attacks. For example, if you suffer from an attack each week, keeping a diary for four to six weeks might be sufficient to notice a pattern emerging. If your attacks are less frequent, you may need to keep a diary for a few months. Note down when each attack happens and then record the details of your daily life at the time that might be relevant. Examples, with suggestions as to what aspects you might consider, include:

**Food** – when and what you ate in the previous 24 hours or so, including whether you missed a meal.

**Drink** – did you drink red wine, or more or less coffee than usual?

**Work patterns** – were you working shifts or overtime?

**Emotions** – were you happy, angry, worried or stressed at any time?

**Sleep** – had you slept for the usual amount of time, or for less time, or more?

**Hormones** – did the migraine occur just before or during menstruation? Are you taking the oral contraceptive pill or HRT?

**Timing** – did the attack happen at the weekend or whilst on holiday?

**Medications** – were you taking medication for another condition at the time of the attack?

Over a period of time you may start to notice a pattern emerging and be able to identify your own particular migraine triggers and other factors in your life that could have lowered your threshold. Some triggers may be beyond your control, such as the weather or your menstrual cycle, but there is plenty you can do about others, including your diet or stress levels. Keeping to regular eating, physical activity, relaxation and sleep routine – even at weekends and during holidays – is one of the best ways of avoiding an attack. In the case of menstrual and menstrually-related migraines, reducing your other triggers and following a healthy lifestyle may be enough to ward off attacks. If not, your GP will be able to prescribe preventative medication or treatments that can abort an attack. See Chapter 5 – Migraine and Hormones for more information.

##  Visit your GP

We've already noted that many migraine sufferers do not bother to visit a GP, often because they have family members with the condition and they believe that nothing can be done. For others, it is because their attacks are so infrequent; I didn't see my GP until my attacks began happening more often. It is a good idea to try to deal with the condition yourself first. You may find that by following the advice in this book, i.e. identifying your triggers, eating healthily, using appropriate natural supplements and over-the-counter medications and managing stress, you can reduce the frequency, length and severity of your attacks and even prevent them. However, there may be times when these strategies are not enough and you need to see your GP. Often in such cases it is more effective to combine natural, preventative strategies with conventional drug treatments. For example, you may manage to get the number of attacks down to a minimum, but still need medication for when a migraine does occur. Also, if you are not quite sure whether you are suffering from migraines, it is a good idea to visit your GP for a definite diagnosis and to rule out any other underlying conditions or more serious health problems.

The most important thing to do when you visit your GP is to make sure you give a full and accurate account of your condition. Research by the Migraine Action Association showed that migraine sufferers often had up to five consultations before their GP demonstrated an understanding of the impact migraines had on their lives. Migraineurs admitted they found it difficult to communicate the extent of their suffering adequately to doctors. So when you visit the surgery it is a good idea to take along a record of when your attacks happened and the symptoms, including their intensity, duration and impact on your life. Include details of medications taken and any possible triggers you have identified. The Migraine Association of Ireland, the National Migraine Centre, The Migraine Trust and McNeil Healthcare (the manufacturers of Migraleve) all offer a downloadable Migraine Diary with columns for recording details like these. The contact details for these organisations can be found in the Directory at the end of the book. This information will help your GP to make a more accurate diagnosis and to prescribe suitable medications, either to help prevent or treat attacks.

For more information about over-the-counter and prescription drugs recommended for the treatment of migraine, see Chapter 7 – Medical and Other Treatments.

Always see a doctor if you have any of these symptoms as they could indicate a more serious problem such as concussion or meningitis:

- You have a headache with drowsiness, nausea, vomiting and light intolerance – especially if it follows a head injury.
- Your headache is accompanied by a stiff neck and a fever.
- You have a persistent headache that is worse in the mornings or is accompanied by sore temples.
- Your headache doesn't respond to self-help treatments within three to seven days.

Chapter 2

# The Food Factor

In this chapter we look at how eating habits, food sensitivities, consumption of particular foods and nutritional status may play a part in triggering migraines.

## 5 Check your caffeine intake

Caffeine can be both a migraine treatment and trigger. If you are not a regular coffee or tea drinker, one cup of strong tea or coffee or a glass of cola can help to abort a migraine, especially when taken in conjunction with medication. Caffeine is thought to constrict the dilated blood vessels around the brain and also maximise the effectiveness of painkillers. Some over-the-counter headache formulations include caffeine as well as an analgesic for this reason.

However, if you regularly drink caffeine-rich drinks and your intake suddenly drops, perhaps after a lie-in at the weekend or simply because you consume less when you're away from the office, the blood vessels around the brain may widen and trigger a migraine.

Paradoxically, drinking too much coffee can trigger migraines. It is thought that overindulgence leads to the blood vessels becoming overly constricted. Drinking a lot of coffee can also lead to peaks and troughs in blood sugar levels, which can lead to migraines in some people. It is also a diuretic, which can lead to dehydration – another factor that can induce a migraine.

Whilst everyone is different, it is thought that drinking more than two cups of coffee or two cans of cola, containing 150–250 mg of caffeine, could be enough to cause problems. If you drink more than this amount, and think caffeine could be implicated in your migraines, it is best to reduce your intake gradually. Try cutting out one cup of coffee, tea or glass of cola daily to avoid a caffeine-withdrawal migraine. Make sure you drink plenty of other fluids, such as water and fruit juices. Another option would be to drink decaffeinated coffee and cola.

If you are a chocolate lover, remember that it also contains caffeine. According to the Food Standards Agency plain chocolate contains the most – around 75 mg per 100 g – and milk chocolate contains about half this amount.

## 6 Watch your blood sugar levels

A drop in blood sugar is a common migraine trigger. Blood sugar levels fluctuate according to food intake and medications;

various hormones are also involved. When blood sugar levels drop too low, hypoglycaemia (low blood sugar) can result. When this happens, the brain doesn't receive sufficient glucose to function properly. The body then reacts by producing hormones that release glucose into the bloodstream. The blood pressure rises as a result and it is thought the diameter of the blood vessels is also affected, leading to a migraine.

One sufferer claims that she can abort a migraine fairly quickly if she eats a piece of cheese and takes two painkillers, such as aspirin or ibuprofen, with either a cup of coffee or a glass of cola at the first signs of an attack. This probably works because the caffeine boosts the painkillers' effects and the cheese raises the blood sugar.

## Go low GI

Missing meals, and eating the wrong types of food, can lead to low blood sugar. Eating regularly – never going longer than four hours without food – and choosing foods with a low Glycaemic Index can help to keep the blood sugar steady. In a survey by the Migraine Action Association, involving 632 people, 270 (43 per cent) said eating regularly helped them to control their migraines.

The Glycaemic Index (GI) is a measure of the rate a food raises the level of sugar in the blood. Refined carbohydrates, such as white bread, pastries, sugary drinks and sweets, convert easily into glucose, causing your blood sugar to rise rapidly, which means they have a high GI. Carbohydrates, such as multigrain bread, porridge, sweet potatoes, pasta, and basmati or brown rice, take longer to digest and cause your blood glucose to rise slowly and remain steady for a longer period of time, because they have a low GI.

For a low GI diet, replace all refined carbohydrates (listed above) with whole grains. Eat plenty of fruit and vegetables, low-fat yogurts and cheeses, and skimmed/semi-skimmed milk. Include small amounts of nuts, fish and lean meat. Leave the skins on potatoes so they take longer to digest. New potatoes, boiled in their skins, have the lowest GI. This type of diet will also help you manage your weight healthily, without resorting to strict dieting, which can trigger migraines, especially if you miss meals in an effort to lose weight. As well as eating regular meals, snacking on fresh fruit, oat cakes or a small handful of nuts or seeds also helps to maintain blood sugar levels.

## 7 Be aware of food intolerances

Another possibility is that migraine is a symptom of a food allergy or intolerance. True food allergy is relatively rare and symptoms are more likely to be due to an intolerance. Food allergy involves an almost immediate, severe response by the immune system after eating a foodstuff. Food intolerance tends to be caused by hypersensitivity to a food. The symptoms tend to be milder and can develop between six and 24 hours later. Common foods linked to intolerance include dairy products, citrus fruits and wheat. Diet may be more important in some sufferers than others. In a survey by the Migraine Association, 189 migraineurs – 41 per cent of 482 respondents – said they'd noticed that eating particular foods could trigger a migraine. Various other foods, drinks and additives are considered to be potential migraine triggers.

## 8 Watch out for tyramine

Tyramine is an amino acid found naturally in certain foods and alcoholic drinks such as red wine and beer. It is thought that some people are more susceptible to the effects of tyramine because they don't have the enzymes to remove it as quickly, which means it remains in the body for longer and could also explain why some migraineurs have shown raised levels. Tyramines are thought to reduce serotonin levels in the brain and thus lead to a narrowing and then widening of the blood vessels. The evidence for a tyramine-migraine link is outdated and inconclusive but, anecdotally, some sufferers claim they find relief when they avoid foods containing it. Foods containing tyramine are usually preserved or aged and include:

- Meat, fish, poultry and eggs – including processed meats, pork, venison and pickled herrings.
- Dairy foods, including cheese – especially aged cheeses like Stilton and blue cheeses, sour cream and yogurt.

- Fruit and vegetables, including citrus fruits (especially oranges), avocados, over-ripe bananas, tomatoes, aubergines.
- Nuts, soya and seeds.
- Vinegar and foods containing vinegar – for example pickles.
- Yeast products, including freshly baked bread and yeast extract.
- Chocolate.

**Chocolate and migraine**

Chocolate often gets the blame for causing migraines, but is it always the culprit? Several studies, in which volunteer migraineurs were given either chocolate or a chocolate substitute called carob, have shown that chocolate was no more likely to trigger an attack than the chocolate substitute.

Migraineurs who ate chocolate and then suffered a migraine could be sensitive to the tyramine or caffeine it contains. However, for some sufferers it could be that craving sweet and sugary foods, such as chocolate, is a prodrome symptom, meaning that rather than being a trigger, eating chocolate is actually a sign that an attack is on its way.

# 9 Be aware of food additives

Additives are used by food manufacturers for various reasons, including to enhance the flavour and colour of food, as well as extend the shelf life and prevent ingredients from separating or clumping together. There's no definitive evidence that they cause migraines, but many migraine sufferers report sensitivity to food additives and this link has been noted by various migraine organisations, including the Migraine Action Association. Although research indicates that food additives are generally safe, some people may find that they are sensitive to specific ones. These are some of the additives that have been linked to migraine:

**Monosodium glutamate (MSG, E621)**

Monosodium glutamate is found naturally in sun-dried tomatoes and Parmesan cheese. It is the sodium salt of glutamic acid and is synthetically produced for use as a flavour enhancer in various foods. It is usually found in soups, broths, flavoured noodles, canned meats and restaurant food, as well as crisps, soy sauce and dry roasted peanuts. Other terms manufacturers use on food labels to indicate its presence include: 'yeast extract', 'hydrolised vegetable protein', 'sodium caseinate', 'texturised protein', 'autolysed yeast' and 'hydrolised oat flour'. It is thought that monosodium glutamate could stimulate nerve cells to release certain brain chemicals that cause changes in the blood vessels in the head and neck and can lead to a migraine.

### Nitrates and Nitrites

Nitrates are not used as widely as in the past. They are naturally occurring minerals and include sodium nitrate and potassium nitrate. The man-made nitrite, sodium nitrite, and naturally occurring potassium nitrite continue to be added to processed meats, including hot dogs, bacon, luncheon meats and pepperoni. Nitrites are used as a preservative as well as to inhibit bacteria and improve the colour and flavour of these foods. Several studies have suggested that nitrites may exacerbate headaches in migraineurs.

### Aspartame

Aspartame is an artificial sweetener made from two amino acids (protein building blocks) – aspartic acid and phenylaline – that has been approved for use and is generally considered safe. It is available on its own, in powder or tablet form, and is also found in diet food products including low calorie fizzy drinks, desserts and chewing gum. Some experts recommend that migraineurs should use it with caution.

### Tartrazine (E102)

This is a yellow dye used to colour some drugs, squashes and fizzy drinks, as well as foods like marzipan and piccalilli sauce. The Migraine Action Association reports that some members claim tartrazine triggers their migraine attacks, but there is no clinical evidence of a link.

### Sulphites

Sulphites are synthetic preservatives used to keep fruits and vegetables looking fresh and are found in alcoholic drinks – especially wines. Sulphites are also used in squashes, pickled onions and red cabbage. Some migraineurs claim that their headaches are triggered by foods containing sulphites, but there's no conclusive evidence of a direct link. Alcohol withdrawal is known to cause headaches and it may be this, rather than sulphites, that triggers migraines.

### Sodium Benzoate

This is an anti-bacterial, anti-fungal preservative derived from benzoic acid. It is effective in foods that are slightly acidic: prawns, margarine, soft drinks, cheesecake mix, soy sauce, orange squash and sweets. There is no clinical evidence of a link with migraines, but the Migraine Action Association reports that some members have identified it as a trigger.

## 10 Keep a food diary

If you feel that particular foods or additives are a factor in your migraine attacks, it may be helpful to keep a food diary to help you identify which, if any, are responsible. When trying to identify food triggers, look at what you ate two to three days beforehand, because a migraine attack actually begins one to two days before you develop the headache – see 'prodrome' in the Introduction. If you suspect a link between a particular food (or food additive) and your migraine attacks, try avoiding or limiting it in your diet and note whether or not your attacks decrease. To avoid food additives, choose unprocessed foods and read food labels. The surest way to identify food triggers is to follow an elimination diet. However, such a diet can lead to nutritional deficiencies and should only be undertaken under medical supervision.

Some experts remain unconvinced of the benefits of avoiding particular foods. Dr MacGregor told me, 'We are keen to minimise the role of specific foods in migraine that always seem to be given such heavy emphasis when the more important message of eating regularly gets lost.'

In an online survey by the Migraine Action Association, in which 812 sufferers took part, only 20 per cent found that food elimination had helped their migraines. On a personal note, I have never been able to link an attack to a particular food, but I have frequently had a migraine after missing a meal or not eating enough.

Another reason why avoiding particular foods and drinks may not reduce the number of attacks is that, as we have already noted, various other factors are usually involved in inducing a migraine. Often, controlling other triggers and eating healthily and regularly can be enough to cut the frequency of attacks.

## 11 Chew ginger

Chewing raw ginger root can ease the nausea and digestive problems that tend to accompany migraines.

Ginger also appears to block the effects of prostaglandins – substances that may cause inflammation of blood vessels in the brain and lead to a migraine. So it may not only ease the nausea associated with migraines, but also help to treat the pain.

If you are not keen on eating raw ginger, try taking it as a tea made by pouring boiling water over three or four thin slices of ginger root and sweetened to taste, preferably with honey. Alternatively, try eating ginger biscuits or crystallised ginger. Ginger biscuits make a good snack to carry around with you to help you deal with an attack.

## 12 Eat magnesium-rich foods

Some studies have suggested that magnesium levels tend to be low in migraineurs. Too little magnesium is thought to lead to a reduced blood flow to the brain and is also linked to low blood sugar. Both of these factors seem to be involved in migraine attacks. Low magnesium levels appear to be especially common in those who suffer from migraine with aura and menstrual migraine. The recommended daily intake is 270 mg for women and 300 mg for men. To ensure an adequate intake of magnesium in your diet, eat plenty of fresh green leafy vegetables, tomato puree, nuts, seeds, wholegrains, beans (including baked beans), peas, potatoes, oats and yeast extract. Avoid drinking too much alcohol; drinking more than the recommended 14 units a week for women and 21 units for men can affect magnesium absorption. Fizzy drinks are also best avoided because the phosphates they contain interfere with magnesium absorption. For more information about magnesium and supplementing your diet with it, see Chapter 3 – Supplementary Benefits.

## 13 Boost your serotonin levels

We've already noted that serotonin affects the blood vessels around the brain and may be implicated in migraine. Also, some studies have shown low levels in migraine sufferers. Serotonin is made in the body from 5HTP (5-hydroxytryptophan), which is produced from L-tryptophan, an amino acid found in protein-rich foods such as chicken, turkey, eggs and dairy foods, as well as bananas, beans, dates, oats, rice, wholegrains, nuts and seeds. Some studies suggest that taking a 5HTP supplement may help to reduce the frequency, severity and length of attacks. See Chapter 3 – Supplementary Benefits for more information.

## 14 Drink water

Dehydration is another common and often overlooked trigger for migraines. The tissues surrounding the brain are composed mainly of water. When these tissues lose fluid, they shrink, leading to irritation and pain.

Some natural health practitioners claim that drinking insufficient water leads to a build up of toxins, which can trigger a migraine in some people – drinking between one and two litres of water daily flushes the whole system and seems to reduce symptoms in some migraineurs.

A small study of 18 migraine sufferers in 2005 found that when half of the participants drank an extra litre of water a day, they reported a reduction in the frequency, duration and severity of attacks. Other studies have linked migraines to drinking insufficient water and some have suggested that drinking half to one litre of water very early on in an attack can help to relieve symptoms. Obviously this would only work if you're dehydrated in the first place.

# Chapter 3

# Supplementary Benefits

There are various herbal, vitamin and mineral supplements that have been recommended for the prevention, or treatment, of migraines. However, it is important to remember that just because something can be termed 'natural' it is not necessarily safe. Also, there is often not enough research and therefore evidence to confirm or disprove claims.

Dr MacGregor told me that she and her then colleagues at the National Migraine Centre were happy to recommend complementary approaches, including supplements like co-enzyme Q10 and butterbur, but cautioned: 'Although controlled clinical trials have shown they are effective in treating migraine, the studies have been short-term, in small numbers of people, and we have no information about long-term effectiveness or, more importantly, about long-term safety.'

## 15 Benefit from supplements

Migraine is an individual condition and what might work for one person may not work for another. If you decide to try any of the supplements mentioned here, it is probably wise to try them for three months and then stop if you do not notice any improvements in your condition. Whilst it is wise to be sceptical of claims of a miraculous cure, there is evidence that many people do benefit from dietary supplements. Remember that herbal remedies are medicines and, like any medicine, may have adverse effects. They may also interact with other medications. Always inform your GP if you are taking herbal medicines or other supplements.

Herbal products are sold as either traditional herbal registration (THR) remedies or herbal food supplements. THR products are regulated and monitored by the government agency known as the Medicines and Healthcare products Regulatory Authority (MHRA). If a product has a THR stamp, it means the MHRA is satisfied that it meets quality standards, has appropriate labelling and a product information leaflet. It also indicates that the herb has been used in traditional remedies for over 30 years. All THR products have a nine-digit registration number starting with the letters THR on the container or packaging.

Herbal food supplements come under the remit of the Food Standards Agency (FSA) and the Chartered Trading Standards Institute at local authority level and are not under the same legal and manufacturing scrutiny. This means there is no guarantee of their content or quality. In 2015, the school of pharmacy at University College London tested over 70 of the most popular herbal remedies bought from the high street or online and found that up to a third contained very little or none of the main ingredient.

There is a full list of herbal medicines granted a traditional herbal registration on the MHRA website as well as further advice and information about using herbal medicines safely. The contact details are in the Directory at the end of this book.

## 5HTP

Taking a supplement of 5-hydroxytryptophan (5HTP) has been shown to reduce the number and severity of migraine attacks in some sufferers. 5HTP is used by the body to make serotonin: a brain chemical that has a role in the regulation of mood, appetite and sleep patterns, as well as other functions including the widening and narrowing of the blood vessels. Research suggests that some migraineurs have low levels of serotonin. One study concluded that sufferers of migraine with aura had significantly lower levels of serotonin than those with migraine without aura, or non-migraineurs, and suggested that this might be due to them having problems metabolising it.

In one study 40 migraine sufferers who took either 200 mg per day of 5HTP, or a drug used to prevent migraines called methysergide, for 40 days found their attacks halved. In two double-blind trials, daily doses of 600 mg of 5HTP were found to be as effective as some medications for reducing migraine attacks in adults. In a double-blind placebo-controlled trial (where one group receives a placebo and another a treatment – both unknowingly), 90 per cent of sufferers taking 400 mg of 5HTP a day found the number, severity and duration of their attacks was reduced.

5HTP supplements are usually derived from the seeds of the griffonia plant found in West Africa. It is recommended that you take 100 mg daily to begin with, increasing to 200–300 mg per day, if required; 5HTP should not be taken with antidepressants (such as Prozac), weight-control drugs or if you're pregnant.

### Coenzyme Q10

A few studies have suggested that taking 150–300 mg of coenzyme daily can help to prevent migraines. Coenzyme Q10 is an element that is both produced by the body and found in foods. It is believed to speed up the metabolic process, helping to provide energy, and is an antioxidant.

One small study of 32 people with a history of migraines (with or without aura) showed that taking a daily dose of 150 mg over a period of three months, on average, more than halved the number of attacks. In addition, 61 per cent of participants found the duration of their attacks was more than halved, while 93 per cent reported the length of their attacks had reduced by a quarter. These results were later confirmed by a double-blind trial using a 300 mg dose. Researchers are unsure how coenzyme Q10 reduces migraines. One theory is that it works by improving the release of energy in the brain cells.

Benefits can be noticed after about four weeks, but it often takes five to 12 weeks before attacks are reduced by up to half.

## Magnesium

In the late 1990s Dr Jay S. Cohen, an expert in prescription drugs and their natural alternatives in the US, found that a magnesium supplement not only successfully treated a problem with the blood vessels in his legs, but also completely cured his migraines. Drawing on studies that suggested that magnesium supplementation could benefit migraine sufferers, he wrote *The Magnesium Solution*.

We have already talked about ensuring you eat magnesium-rich foods, because insufficient magnesium can lead to reduced blood flow to the brain. Research suggests that magnesium helps to regulate the size of blood vessels in the brain and reduces the risk of them constricting (narrowing) or dilating (widening), so that the blood flow remains stable. It also appears to keep the nervous system functioning normally – as we've already mentioned in the Introduction, the vascular (blood vessel) and nervous systems are thought to be involved in migraine. Magnesium is also thought to reduce blood clotting and have anti-inflammatory properties, which may also help to prevent attacks.

Dr Cohen recommends that women take up to 320 mg a day and men 420 mg. He suggests starting with 100 mg twice daily and increasing the dose gradually to help avoid gastrointestinal upsets.

**Note**

If you have high blood pressure, heart or kidney problems, see your GP before supplementing with magnesium.

## Feverfew

The herb feverfew has been taken for the relief of headaches since the seventeenth century. A member of the sunflower family, it has small, daisy-like flowers and is common in Europe, Canada and North America. Over the years people have claimed that after taking feverfew for a while, they've suffered fewer migraine attacks or, in some cases, that their attacks have stopped completely.

A well-designed study in 2005 provided scientific evidence that feverfew can help to prevent migraines. The study used freeze-dried capsules, but you can also buy feverfew in tablet form. A daily dose of 250 mg is recommended. Alternatively, you can grow your own plant and either eat the fresh leaves or dry them to make your own herbal tea. The leaves are quite bitter, so one of the most palatable ways of eating them is in a feverfew and honey sandwich. The suggested number of leaves is one large leaf (approx 12 cm long) or three small leaves (approx 4 cm). You can also dry the leaves and store them in a jar until you are ready to use them. Using the same quantity as for the sandwich, place them in a cup, add boiling water and leave to infuse for a few minutes before removing the leaves and drinking. Again, because of the bitter flavour, adding honey can make the tea more pleasant to drink.

Feverfew only works when taken as a preventative, it does not help to relieve a migraine once it is under way. Researchers are unsure which constituents of feverfew exert the beneficial effects. Some suggest it is a substance called parthenolide, which has anti-inflammatory properties and may affect serotonin levels. Others believe it is the high melatonin content which has a preventative effect, or possibly the pain-relieving effects of an essential oil contained in the plant.

Researchers claim that side effects from feverfew are generally mild. Some people find direct contact with feverfew leaves causes dermatitis and irritates the mouth – sometimes leading to ulcers. It may also cause stomach upsets in some users.

It is not recommended during pregnancy as it may cause contractions. Also, if you take aspirin regularly, see your GP before using this herb as it has similar blood-thinning properties.

If you want to stop taking feverfew, try to do so gradually as some users have found that stopping abruptly led to the return of their migraines, along with other symptoms like nausea, insomnia and anxiety.

## Vitamin B2 (riboflavin)

There is evidence that 400 mg of vitamin B2 daily can act as a preventative in migraine. Some studies suggested that the number of attacks experienced by migraineurs halved within three to four months.

### Triple therapy

A leading US migraine expert, Dr Alexander Mauskop, recommends taking 100 mg of feverfew, 300–400 mg of magnesium and 400 mg of riboflavin daily. A product called MigreLief is available that provides this combination in the right proportions. Further details can be found in the Useful Products section.

## Vitamin B3 (niacin)

The well-known nutritional therapist Patrick Holford recommends taking 100–200 mg of vitamin B3 at the first sign of a migraine. He claims that vitamin B3 is a vasodilator, which means it opens up the blood vessels, and that it can often stop or reduce migraine symptoms. You may experience flushing or a feeling of heat. He also recommends taking vitamin B3 to prevent attacks, saying there is evidence that taking 100 mg daily can halve the number of attacks. If you prefer to obtain this vitamin from your food, include beef, pork, chicken, fish, nuts, dairy foods, wheat flour, potatoes and pasta in your diet as they are all good sources.

## Other B vitamins

Patrick Holford also claims that taking other B vitamins (e.g. B6, B12 and folic acid) may help migraine sufferers because they have been shown to lower homocysteine levels in the body. This is thought to be because they are involved in the breaking down of homocysteine. Homocysteine is an amino acid produced by the body that has an effect on the blood vessels; high levels in the body have been linked to stroke and heart disease. Some studies have also linked these raised levels to migraine attacks – especially those with aura. One study in particular linked the overproduction of homocysteine with a genetic mutation which it claimed was twice as common in migraine sufferers and four times as common among those who experienced migraine with aura. The design of some of these studies has been called into question, but nonetheless they might at least partly explain why, for many people, the tendency to suffer from migraines seems to be inherited and why some B vitamins appear to be beneficial.

Interestingly, in her book *Let's Eat Right to Keep Fit*, published almost 40 years ago, the late renowned American nutritionist Adelle Davis claimed that migraines often cleared up with adequate vitamin B6, and that a lack of vitamin B1 and niacin (B3) was linked to the condition.

## Calcium

Adelle Davis also stated in *Let's Eat Right to Keep Fit* that migraine sufferers would benefit most from taking calcium as well as vitamin B6. This is an interesting idea because one of the theories as to why Topamax, the anti-epilepsy drug, appears to help migraine is that it increases calcium levels. Davis also believed that calcium levels in women were linked to hormone levels, suggesting that the dip in oestrogen around the time of menstruation corresponded to a drop in calcium, which was responsible for premenstrual symptoms, such as irritability and depression. Many women suffer from migraine around the time of menstruation, so perhaps low calcium levels could be implicated.

There is some evidence that a calcium and vitamin-D-rich diet helps to ease PMT symptoms. The 2007 BBC series *The Truth About Food* reported on a three-month trial at the Queen Charlotte Hospital, London, involving 16 women suffering from PMT. Half of the women were given a placebo pill and senior nutritionist Nigel Denby asked the other half to eat foods rich in calcium (such as low fat milk, cheese and yogurt) along with oily fish (such as salmon, mackerel and herring) for vitamin D to aid the absorption of calcium. The women were asked to rate their symptoms before the trial and then to keep a diary recording their symptoms each day during it. According to consultant gynaecologist Dr Nick Panay, those on the 'Double D' diet showed a reduction in symptoms of around a third.

## Fish oils

Studies in Greenland noted that few Inuits suffered from migraines. The Inuits' diet is rich in omega 3 fatty acids, because they eat a lot of fish and the meat and fat from sea mammals.

Two uncontrolled pilot studies were carried out to try to find out whether fish oils could benefit migraine sufferers. One study in Sweden involving 41 people, of whom 33 suffered more than one attack per week and eight had less frequent attacks, suggested that fish oils may help both to prevent migraine attacks and reduce their severity. After taking an omega 3 supplement for three months, those with the most frequent attacks experienced 28 per cent fewer attacks and a 32 per cent reduction in their severity. The results of a questionnaire indicated that 67 per cent of those with the most frequent attacks felt their quality of life had improved. Sixty-three per cent of those with fewer attacks noted an improvement.

A similar Danish trial involved 35 migraineurs – 21 with frequent attacks and 14 with fewer. Those in the first group showed a 57 per cent reduction in both the severity and frequency of their attacks. The second group reported 43 per cent fewer migraines and a 36 per cent reduction in intensity.

Whilst the results were positive, these were short-term uncontrolled studies – which means there was no comparison group – so the evidence is inconclusive. However, omega 3 oils are believed to be anti-inflammatory and research suggests they are essential for healthy brain function. They are also involved in the production of prostaglandins, which are hormone-like substances that regulate the expansion and narrowing of blood vessels, so they may be worth trying as a preventative treatment. The British Dietetic Association suggests supplementing daily with 450–900 mg of omega 3 oils – roughly the amount provided by two to four portions of oily fish.

**Note**

Omega 3 oils have an anti-clotting effect, so avoid taking them if you are on warfarin. If you are pregnant, avoid taking fish liver oils such as cod liver oil, as they're also high in vitamin A. Too much vitamin A can harm your unborn baby. Fish oil supplements (often labelled omega 3 supplements) are safe to take while pregnant.

### Glucosamine

Glucosamine is an essential building block of joint cartilage, ligaments, bone and blood vessels and is a natural substance that your body produces. Glucosamine seems to slow down the degeneration of cartilage and is anti-inflammatory. Clinical trials have shown that glucosamine supplementation can both relieve symptoms and slow the progression of osteoarthritis.

These results prompted further research to see whether it could help other conditions. One study suggested that it may improve migraines. But the trial involved only ten people over a period of just four to six weeks, so further research is needed to confirm whether or not glucosamine supplementation is beneficial for migraineurs. If you want to try it, the suggested dose is 1,500–2,000 mg a day.

### Melatonin

Recent research suggests that melatonin may help to prevent migraines. Melatonin is the hormone that regulates the sleep-wake cycle and is produced in response to light by the pineal gland in the brain. Considering that too much or too little sleep are common migraine triggers, it seems sensible to assume that melatonin may play a part in migraine. Melatonin is also involved in stabilising the blood vessels in the brain and is anti-inflammatory. It is thought that too little melatonin in the body may be linked to migraines and cluster headaches. Research has shown that migraineurs often have low levels and our bodies also produce less as we get older.

A small study by Brazilian scientists in 2004 involved 34 migraine patients suffering between two and eight migraine attacks, with or without aura, a month. Twenty-nine of the participants were women. The participants took no melatonin in the first month and then took 3 mg of melatonin each day for three months, half an hour before bedtime.

After taking melatonin for three months, over two-thirds of the participants reported that the number of migraines they experienced was cut by half, or more. Some noticed benefits before the end of the three-month trial. A further randomised, double-blind placebo-controlled study by the same researchers in 2013 concluded that 3 mg of melatonin taken between 10 p.m. and 11 p.m. every night is as effective as amitriptyline in reducing migraine frequency and has fewer side-effects.

Interestingly, serotonin is used by the body to make melatonin, and we have already noted how this brain chemical appears to benefit some migraineurs. We have also seen how changes in sleep patterns can be a trigger for migraines.

Melatonin can be bought over-the-counter as a supplement (see Useful Products) and is also prescribed for insomnia in people aged over 55. If side effects are experienced, they are usually mild; however, if you are taking medication speak to your GP before taking melatonin as it can interact with certain ones – including blood-thinners (anticoagulants), immunosuppressants, diabetes medications and birth control pills.

You can encourage your body to produce more melatonin by eating foods rich in tryptophan, which the body uses to make serotonin (see Boost your serotonin levels in chapter 2). Another way to boost melatonin production is to get out in natural light during the day.

# Chapter 4

# Mind Over Migraine

We have already noted that stress can be an important factor in migraine headaches. Research has shown that stress management and relaxation can help in migraine prevention. In this chapter we look at what stress is, as well as the symptoms and causes. We also identify techniques that could help you deal with stress better and relax, including changing your attitude, deep breathing and even just having a good laugh.

Although some migraine sufferers become indignant when anyone suggests that some aspects of their personality could contribute to their attacks, I have explored this idea, because I think some people may find an element of truth in it. We also look at a suggestion from a leading neurologist that, in some people, a migraine attack may even serve a purpose – like helping the mind or body to recover from stress, or even as a way of expressing repressed emotions. This chapter also includes tips to help you sleep better and be more assertive.

## What is stress?

Stress is basically how the mind and body respond to pressures, such as unforeseen events or excessive demands in our working and home lives, that leave us feeling inadequate or unable to cope. One person may adapt well to a situation that another may find stressful. It's all down to the individual's perception of it and their ability to deal with it.

Your brain reacts to stress by preparing the body either to face the perceived threat or to escape from it. It does this by releasing hormones – chemical messengers – including adrenaline, noradrenaline and cortisol, into the bloodstream. These speed up the heart rate and breathing patterns and may induce sweating. Glucose and fatty acid levels in the blood rise, providing a burst of energy to enable you to deal with the threat or run away from it. This is called the 'fight or flight' response.

These days stressful situations, such as pressure at work, or a life changing event, like bereavement or redundancy, are ongoing and unlikely to necessitate or be alleviated by either of these abrupt reactions, so stress hormone levels are likely to remain high. Over time, these chemicals can have a detrimental effect on health, leading to an increased risk of major health problems, such as coronary heart disease, as well as psychosomatic disorders (involving both mind and body), including migraines. Many people are living increasingly busy lives, so it is important to find ways of recognising, reducing and managing stress.

### Recognise stress

It is important to recognise the physical symptoms of stress as soon as they arise, so that you can take action before you suffer any health problems.

Common psychological signs of stress include:

- Anxiety, depression, low self-esteem or apathy.
- Poor concentration, poor short-term memory or indecisiveness.
- Irrational or rash decision-making, irritability or anger.
- Tearfulness, loss of appetite (possibly leading to low blood sugar – a migraine trigger), or comfort eating, smoking, drinking or using recreational drugs.
- Difficulty in completing simple tasks, feeling disorganised, poor co-ordination.

Common physical signs of stress include:

- Tension in the jaws, shoulders and neck. General aches and pains – due to muscle tension.
- Headaches – including migraines.
- Skin problems, such as eczema.
- Fidgeting, sweating, a dry mouth.
- Exhaustion, stomach ache, nausea.
- Diarrhoea, increased urination, difficulty sleeping.
- Weight gain, or weight loss.
- Increased infections – due to reduced immunity.
- Heart palpitations, breathlessness, missed periods in women.

## Migraine and stress release

Some people find they suffer from more migraines on a Saturday morning, which is when they start to relax at the end of their working week, or at other times when stress is released, for example on holiday. The best solution is to try to avoid a build up of stress during your working week by regularly taking time out to relax and using other stress management techniques, such as those outlined in this chapter.

## Other possible triggers

### Heightened sensitivity

A heightened sensitivity to light, noise and smell is a common symptom of migraines. Dr Peter Goadsby, a professor of clinical neurology who works with The Migraine Trust, has suggested that migraineurs may regularly be in a state of heightened perception and this may at times overcharge, leading to an attack.

### Psychological approaches

In his classic book *Migraine*, the late neurologist Dr Oliver Sacks looked at various psychological theories surrounding migraine and suggested that, in some sufferers, their condition may actually serve a purpose. I think this is an interesting alternative view on migraines that's worth considering when trying to find out what triggers your attacks.

### Migraines as recuperation

Dr Sacks pointed out that when migraines occur after a prolonged period of emotional or physical activity, they could be viewed as recuperative, because the sufferer is usually forced to rest until the attack has passed. He noted that such people are often full of renewed energy after an attack.

Could migraine be the body's way of forcing those with a driven and obsessive personality to ease up? Although I've linked my own attacks with hormonal factors and missing meals, I can still identify with this idea: I have often suffered from an attack at the weekend, whilst on holiday or after an especially busy or stressful time.

## Expression of repression

Dr Sacks also put forward the idea that, in some sufferers, migraines may serve as a way of expressing repressed emotions – especially anger and hostility. This is another interesting theory, since women generally have more problems in expressing anger than men, and they tend to suffer from migraines more often than men.

### Is there a migraine personality?

One popular theory to explain why some people suffer from migraines suggests that particular personality types are more predisposed to the condition – usually type A personalities who tend to be ambitious, competitive and impatient. Yet lots of migraine sufferers would argue that they are not like that at all and plenty of people with those personality traits don't suffer from migraines. However, if you've inherited a tendency to suffer from migraines, having a type A personality could mean you lead a more stressful lifestyle and prolonged stress does seem to be a migraine trigger for many sufferers.

## 16 Identify your stress triggers

For a couple of weeks record the details of situations, times, places and people that make you feel stressed. Once you've identified your stressors, you can find ways to avoid, minimise or learn to deal with them better. Some stress-busting techniques include the following:

### Don't sweat the small stuff!

As well as recognising the external factors that make you feel stressed, consider whether some aspects of your personality are also to blame. Are you a perfectionist who is never satisfied with your achievements and lifestyle? Constantly feeling that who you are, and what you have, is not good enough, can lead to unrealistic expectations, discontent and unnecessary pressure. In his best-selling book *Don't Sweat the Small Stuff*, the late Dr Richard Carlson urged us to remind ourselves that 'life is okay the way it is, right now.' Adopting this attitude immediately reduces stress and induces calm.

### Your 'in basket' is never empty!

Workaholism is another stressor that tends to be linked with perfectionism – a 'perfect' home and lifestyle have to be paid for. And whilst working hard for what you want in life is commendable, some people work such long hours they don't have time to enjoy what they have. If you are constantly driven to get everything done and think you will feel calm and relaxed once everything on your 'to do list' is completed, think again! What tends to happen is that new things are added to the list all the time so your 'in basket' is never empty. Dr Carlson used to control his obsession with completing his 'to do lists' by reminding himself that 'the purpose of life isn't to get it all done but to enjoy each step along the way.' He also suggests, 'Remind yourself that when you die, your "in basket" won't be empty.'

## 17 Learn to delegate

Perfectionism can also lead to a need to control – you convince yourself that no one else can meet your high standards and do everything yourself. This inevitably leads to physical and mental overload. The solution is to accept that you can't 'know' and 'do' everything so you need to learn to listen to other people's ideas and opinions and to delegate.

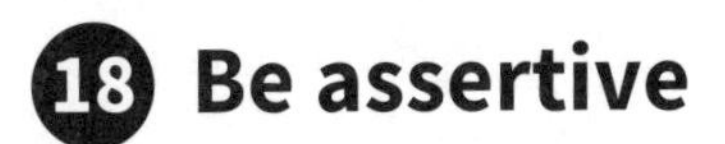

## 18 Be assertive

'No' is a little word that can reduce your stress levels dramatically. If you feel overloaded and your stress levels are rising as a result, try saying ' no' to the non-essential tasks you don't have time for, or just do not want to do. If you find it hard to say 'no', then perhaps you need to improve your assertiveness skills.

## Assert yourself!

If you feel that you often hide your true feelings rather than express them and give in to others so as not to hurt or upset them or to gain their approval, you might benefit from brushing up on your assertiveness skills.

Perhaps you regularly allow others to manipulate you into doing things you do not want to do? Being assertive enables you to say what you want, feel and need, calmly and confidently, without being aggressive or hurting others. Try the following techniques to develop your self-assertiveness so that you remain in control of your life and do things because you want to, rather than to please other people.

- Show ownership of your thoughts, feelings and behaviour by using 'I' rather than 'we', 'you' or 'it'. Instead of saying 'You make me angry', try 'I feel angry when you...' This is also less antagonising to the other person.
- When you have a choice whether to do something or not, say 'won't' rather than 'can't', 'choose to' instead of 'have to' and 'could' rather than 'should' to indicate that you have made an active decision, rather than suggesting that something or someone has stopped you.
- When you feel your needs aren't being addressed, state what you want calmly and clearly, repeating it until the other person shows they hear and understand what you're saying.

- When making a request, identify exactly what you want and what you're prepared to settle for. Choose positive, assertive words, as outlined above.
- When refusing a request, speak calmly but firmly, giving the reason or reasons why, without apologising. Repeat if you need to.
- When you disagree with someone, say so using the word 'I'. Explain why you disagree, whilst acknowledging the other person's right to hold a different viewpoint.

## 19 Accept what you can't change

The Serenity Prayer suggests we should accept the things we can't change, have the courage to change the things we can and have the wisdom to know the difference. This does not mean you should give up and accept that nothing in your life can be changed. It's about not wasting your time and energy worrying about things over which you have no influence or control so that you can focus your efforts where you can make a difference.

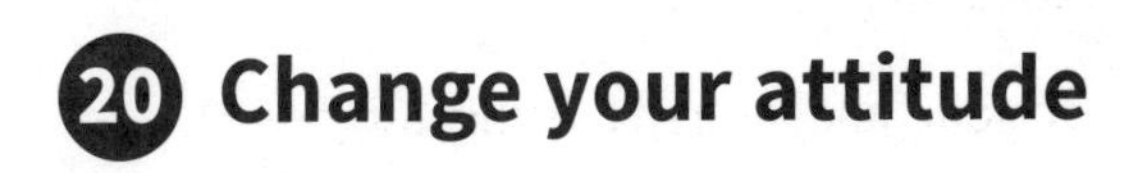

## 20 Change your attitude

Changing your attitude towards situations can reduce stress. When something bad happens, instead of thinking about how awful the situation is, try to find something positive about it if you can. Try to find answers to your problems, or view them as an opportunity for personal growth. For example, being made redundant initially seems like a negative event but, if you view it as an opportunity to retrain and start a new career doing something you really enjoy, it can become a catalyst for positive change.

## 21 Manage your time

If you regularly feel under pressure and stressed due to a lack of time, try reviewing how you use it. Keep a diary for a few days to see how you spend your time and then decide which activities you can cut out, or reduce, to make more time for the things that are most important to you.

**Prioritise**

When you have a long 'to do' list, number tasks in terms of urgency and importance and carry them out in that order.

## 22 Get moving

Regular exercise is a great antidote to stress because it enables the body to utilise the stress hormones whose original purpose was to provide the extra energy needed to run away from our aggressors, or to stay put and fight. It also triggers the release of endorphins, which improve mood and heighten feelings of well-being. Research also suggests that moderate exercise helps to reduce the frequency of migraine attacks.

You do not need to join a gym to become more active, incorporating exercise into your daily routine is easy and effective. Putting more effort into the housework, gardening, walking the dog, getting up from your desk and walking around regularly, walking whilst talking on a mobile, are all ways of being more active. However, do not overdo it; over-exercising can be a migraine trigger. Also, exercise leads to more calories being burnt, so you may need to eat more to avoid your blood sugar levels falling and triggering an attack.

## 23 Go back to nature

Researchers at Essex University say that engaging with nature offers both mental and physical health benefits. Whether through an active pursuit, such as walking or gardening, or a passive one, like admiring the view, being close to nature has been shown to reduce stress and ease muscular tension. Experts believe that the higher levels of negative ions near areas with running water, trees and mountains may play a part. Others claim it's down to 'biophilia': the theory that we have an innate affinity with nature and that our 'disconnection' from it is the cause of stress and mental health problems. Studies in the Netherlands and Japan suggest that people living in or near 'green' areas enjoy a longer and healthier life than those living in urban environments.

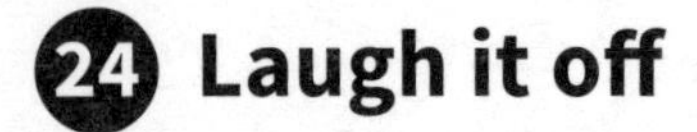

## 24 Laugh it off

Laughter is a great stress reliever. A good belly-laugh seems to reduce the stress hormones cortisol and adrenaline and increase mood-boosting serotonin levels. People who see the funny side of life appear to have a reduced risk of the health problems associated with stress. So make time to watch your favourite comedies and be around people who make you laugh. Or visit www.laughlab.co.uk or www.ahajokes.com whenever you feel like a good giggle.

**Have a hug**

Research suggests that having a regular hug reduces stress hormones in the bloodstream and lowers blood pressure.

## 25 Share problems

Research suggests that people with a good social network tend to have better mental health than those without close friendships. Talking to family members and friends you can trust, when you feel under pressure, can help you to deal with stress.

## 26 Breathe deeply

When you are stressed, your breathing tends to become shallow, or you might hold your breath without realising it.

Slow, deep breathing has been shown to reduce the heart rate, relax muscles and release tension. So next time you're feeling stressed, try taking control of your breathing. Inhale slowly through your nostrils to a count of five, allowing your tummy to expand, hold for a count of five and then breathe out slowly through your nose to a count of five, whilst slowly flattening your stomach. Repeat up to ten times.

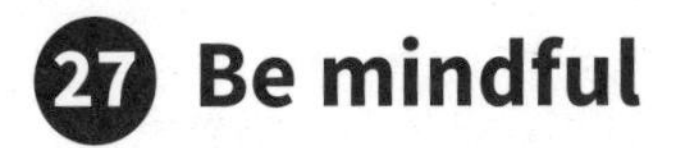

## 27 Be mindful

Mindfulness, stemming from Buddhism, has been shown to reduce stress levels. It involves concentrating on the present, rather than regretting the past or worrying about the future. It is based on the idea that we are not able to change what has already happened or predict the future, but we can influence what is happening now. By focusing fully on the present, you can carry out tasks more efficiently and get the most out of each moment.

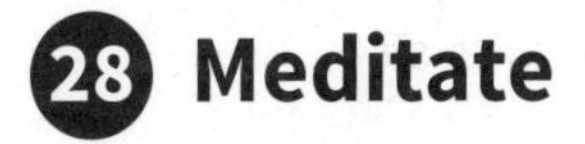

## 28 Meditate

Research suggests that meditation not only lowers stress hormones, but also increases blood flow to the brain. Since migraine is associated with both stress and possibly the constriction of the blood vessels surrounding the brain, it is not surprising that some studies show that meditation can reduce the number of migraines suffered. There are various meditation techniques, but here is a simple one that can be practised whenever you have a few moments to yourself – even whilst on the bus or train!

Close your eyes and focus on your breathing. As you inhale slowly and deeply through your nose, expand your stomach, hold for a few seconds, before drawing in your stomach, whilst exhaling slowly. Whenever your attention is distracted by a passing thought, return to simply observing your breathing.

## 29 Sleep soundly

Sleep is a factor in migraines – too much, or too little, can act as a trigger. Insufficient sleep is also known to increase stress levels.

To enjoy sound sleep, try the following:

- Get outside during the day. Exposure to daylight stops the production of melatonin, the brain chemical that promotes sleep, making it easier for your body to release it at night, so that you drop off more easily and sleep more deeply.
- Ensure your bedroom is cool and dark. Your brain tries to reduce your body temperature at night to slow down your metabolism. So to encourage sleep, aim for a temperature of around 16°C. Darkness stimulates the pineal gland in the brain to produce melatonin.

- To help your brain to associate the bedroom with sleep and sex only, avoid having a TV or computer in your bedroom. Watching TV or using a computer last thing at night may overstimulate your brain, making it harder for you to switch off and fall asleep. Also, both TV and computer screens emit bright light, which may inhibit the production of melatonin.
- Don't drink coffee or cola after 6 p.m. because the stimulant effects of the caffeine they contain can last for hours. Whilst tea contains about half as much caffeine – around 50 mg per cup – it is best not to overdo it near bedtime if you have difficulty sleeping. Redbush tea, which is caffeine-free, makes a good alternative.
- Avoid drinking alcohol at bedtime; it may relax you at first and help you fall asleep more quickly, but its stimulant effect can cause you to wake more during the night. It is also a diuretic, making nocturnal trips to the toilet more likely. But, if abstinence does not help you sleep better, it may be worth indulging in a glass of Cabernet Sauvignon, Merlot or Chianti at bedtime – there is evidence these wines improve your sleep patterns because the grape skins they contain are rich in melatonin. Bear in mind, however, that red wine contains tyramine, which can be a migraine trigger for some sufferers.
- Exercise can help you sleep more soundly, because it encourages your body temperature and metabolism to increase and then fall a few hours later, which promotes

sleep. Try not to exercise later than early evening to benefit. Exercising too late at night may have the opposite effect, because the body temperature may still be raised at bedtime. Lack of exercise can cause sleep problems and restlessness.

- Choose foods rich in tryptophan, an amino acid your body uses to produce serotonin – a brain chemical that is converted into the 'sleep hormone' melatonin. Tryptophan-rich foods include bananas, chicken, turkey, dates, rice, oats, wholegrain breads and cereals. Make sure you are neither too hungry, nor too full when you go to bed, as either can cause wakefulness.
- Soak in a warm bath at bedtime. Your temperature increases slightly with the warmth and then falls – helping you to drop off. Add a few drops of essential oils such as lavender or camomile for their soothing properties.
- If worrying about problems or a busy schedule the next day stops you from falling asleep, try writing down your concerns or a plan for the day before you go to bed.

## 30 Eat a de-stress diet

What you eat also affects your mood and can heighten, or lower, the stress response.

A balanced diet is essential for good mental as well as physical health. Your food intake should be around one third fruit and vegetables, one third carbohydrates (preferably wholegrain), with the remaining third consisting of low fat dairy and protein foods, such as pulses, white fish, lean meat and skinless chicken, and much smaller amounts of fatty and sugary foods. Ensure you have an adequate intake of essential fatty acids by eating oily fish, nuts and seeds and using oils such as flaxseed oil (as a salad dressing) and olive oil (for cooking and as a salad dressing) . This type of diet helps the body to deal more efficiently with stress.

Cutting down on caffeine, alcohol, sugar, salt, refined carbohydrates, saturated and trans fats and highly processed foods enables the mind and body to function more efficiently, without stressful peaks and troughs in energy and mood. We've already seen how coffee and alcohol are sometimes implicated in migraines in other ways so cutting back on these will offer a number of benefits.

## 31 Try natural therapies

Various natural therapies, including acupressure, aromatherapy, massage reflexology and yoga are thought to help relieve psychological stress and muscle tension. For ideas on how you can practise these therapies at home, see Chapter 8 – DIY Complementary Therapies.

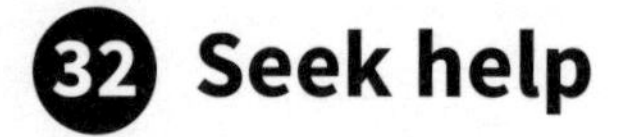

## 32 Seek help

Finally, don't be afraid to ask for professional help if you feel you can't deal with life's stresses on your own. Your first port of call should be your GP, as they will be able to offer advice and possibly refer you to a counsellor.

The International Stress Awareness Association offers further guidance on dealing with stress and referrals to stress management professionals. The Relaxation for Living Institute offers a network of teachers delivering classes to help people to relax and manage their stress levels. The website offers self-help tips to aid relaxation and stress management, details of classes near you and a *Relaxation for Living* DVD. You can find the contact details for all of these groups in the Directory at the end of the book.

**How a 'desperate housewife' de-stresses**

Actress Marcia Cross, who plays Bree Van De Kamp in the TV drama *Desperate Housewives*, said that she reduced the number of classical migraines she suffers to about three or four a year by avoiding certain foods and keeping an eye on her stress levels. She noticed that she often developed a migraine after a particularly stressful period and says she now does not let that happen. She suggests it is helpful to be 'at peace with your own day and your own situation,' and finds yoga and hiking help her to manage her stress levels.

Chapter 5

# Migraine and Hormones

It has long been noted that far more women than men experience migraines. Studies suggest that fluctuations in the female hormone oestrogen may be involved.

## 33 Learn how hormone fluctuations can affect migraines

### Migraines: the menstrual cycle

Research suggests that around half of women who suffer from migraines have noticed a link between migraine attacks and their periods. A survey by the Migraine Action Association in 2005 noted that 73 per cent of women could predict when migraines would occur each month due to their menstrual cycle. These women tended to suffer from an attack either two days before or two days after the start of a period. Many find that these migraines last longer, are more intense and respond less well to treatment than those not linked to periods. It is thought the drop in oestrogen levels that occurs at this time in a woman's cycle is to blame, and some women are especially sensitive to these fluctuations. This may be because oestrogen interacts with serotonin.

A study in 2004 of 155 women over the course of a combined 693 menstrual cycles confirmed that migraines during menstruation were more likely to be severe and linked with nausea and vomiting, compared to attacks at other times during the cycle. Migraine attacks almost doubled in the two days before a period and were twice as severe. Attacks more than doubled in the first three days of a period and their severity more than tripled. Migraines at this time were also five times more likely to lead to vomiting.

Dr MacGregor defines menstrual migraine (pure menstrual migraine) as 'A migraine without aura, occurring only between two days before and three days after the start of a period, over at least two or three cycles.'

In menstrually-related migraine (MRM), migraines without auras occur not only between two days before and three days after a period, but also at other times in the menstrual cycle. Again, migraine attacks are likely to be linked to hormonal fluctuations. It may help to keep a diary, so that after a number of months you can check whether there is a link between attacks and particular times in your cycle. This information will be useful if you need to see your GP about your symptoms. Treatment for the onset of an attack, such as painkillers or triptans, may be effective. Or your GP may suggest one or a combination of preventative treatments for menstrual migraine outlined in this section.

## Migraines: the pill

Many women find that taking an oral contraceptive makes their migraines worse, though a few note an improvement in their symptoms. Taking a 'continuous' contraceptive pill could be beneficial as it keeps hormone levels more stable and prevents the drop in oestrogen that seems to trigger migraines in some women. Oestrogen only, in gel form, or the progestogen only pill may benefit some women. Women who suffer from classical migraines (migraine with aura) shouldn't take an oral contraceptive, because it is thought it may increase the risk of a stroke. Similarly, if you take the pill and develop classical migraine symptoms, you should see your GP immediately to seek an alternative form of contraception.

## Migraines: pregnancy

As with other times of hormonal change, pregnancy can either improve or worsen symptoms. Often migraine attacks may increase in intensity during the first three months of pregnancy. After that about 70 per cent of women notice an improvement. The remaining 30 per cent may experience no change, or a worsening of symptoms. Some women have their first migraine attack during pregnancy or their first migraine with aura. Some women are especially prone to attacks after giving birth, possibly because this is a phase when they're likely to experience various triggers, such as lack of sleep, missed meals, stress, etc. Generally, after pregnancy migraines return to the same type and patterns as before.

The choice of medications for migraine treatment during pregnancy is limited, for obvious reasons, so it is especially important to look after your health and avoid your particular triggers. Rather than taking supplements, try eating a balanced diet containing magnesium and vitamin B2-rich foods (see Chapter 2 – The Food Factor). Paracetamol is a safe form of pain relief during pregnancy, should you need it. If you have frequent attacks that necessitate preventative treatments, see your GP, as they will be able to prescribe a drug that is deemed safe for use during pregnancy.

Feverfew isn't recommended for use during pregnancy, as it may cause contractions.

## Migraines: menopause

Nearly half of female migraine sufferers find their symptoms worsen during the perimenopause – the time leading up to the menopause – this is most likely because the ovaries begin to produce less oestrogen. Another contributing factor could be the changes in sleep patterns that often accompany the perimenopause as a result of night sweats.

## Migraines: HRT

There appears to be no evidence that HRT increases the risk of strokes in women suffering from migraines with auras, but some women may find it makes the condition worse. However, as in the case of the pill, a few women may find their symptoms improve whilst taking HRT. The general advice is to take HRT if you feel your menopausal symptoms warrant it and there are no other contraindications, but to consider stopping taking it if your migraines increase in number and/or severity. It's advisable to discuss your best course of action with your GP.

If your GP suspects that your increased migraines are due to low oestrogen levels, they may reduce the dose. If fluctuations in oestrogen could be to blame, HRT in patch form may be suggested, as it delivers a more steady level of the hormone. The results of a survey conducted by the Migraine Action Association suggested that oestrogen in tablet form was associated with a worsening of migraines, and non-oral routes (patches or gel) were associated with improvement.

If your migraines appear to be triggered by reduced oestrogen levels, your GP may advise you to take continuous combined HRT instead of cyclical combined HRT (HRT in patch form), so that your oestrogen levels remain more constant. If it seems that your migraines may be linked to progestogen, your GP may suggest a change in the type of progestogen you take, or a switch to an HRT patch. It is important to note that continuous combined HRT is only suitable for women who haven't had a period for 12 months or more, as this reduces the risk of irregular bleeding when starting HRT.

## 34 Hormones: keep a diary

The easiest way to detect whether your migraines are hormone related is to keep a diary over at least three cycles. Mark the days of your period with a tick and then indicate each day of a migraine with a cross. If you note a cross on the first ticked day, or two days before or after, it is very likely you are suffering from menstrual migraine. You can take this diary with you when you visit your GP; it will help with the diagnosis.

## 35 Hormones: be prepared

If you suffer from menstrual migraine, what can you do? Try to be prepared. Make sure you have your medication to hand and try to avoid other triggers, such as lack of food, sleep or stress, etc. Try to reduce your workload and commitments around this time. A supplement that is helpful for pre-menstrual symptoms, such as agnus castus or evening primrose oil, may be worth trying. Dr Mauskop recommends a magnesium supplement for menstrual migraine. Also, eating the 'Double D Diet' (as described in Chapter 2 – The Food Factor), which is rich in dairy foods and oily fish, to supply calcium and vitamin D, could help to reduce PMT and therefore reduce attacks. Calcium levels appear to drop at menstruation, and low calcium levels have been linked to migraines, so this could help to partly explain menstrual migraines. If you do not like, or are intolerant to, dairy foods or oily fish, try supplementing your diet with a calcium and vitamin D supplement.

## 36 Choose medications for menstrual migraine

Once your GP has confirmed that you suffer from menstrual migraine, there are various treatment options. For preventative treatments to work, your periods need to be regular and your migraine onset predictable. Preventative treatments include:

### Naproxen

Naproxen is a non-steroidal anti-inflammatory drug (NSAID) that is effective in preventing migraines and relieving menstrual pain.

### Triptans

Used as a preventative rather than as an acute treatment (as they are normally used). Triptans work by balancing serotonin levels in the brain. When used in this way you will need to take them for five days, starting two to three days before the date either your period or migraine is expected – depending which triptan you are prescribed. For more detailed information about triptans, see Chapter 7 – Medical and Other Treatments.

# Chapter 6

# Tackling Other Triggers

This chapter looks at solutions to other common migraine triggers, including changes in sleep patterns, the weather, and neck and shoulder pain.

## 37 Establish a sleep routine

A survey of 143 migraineurs conducted by the Anglo-European College of Chiropractic indicated that 61 per cent felt that their sleep patterns were involved in their attacks. Fifty-one per cent thought that not getting enough sleep was a trigger for their migraines, whilst 36 per cent thought that too much sleep was a factor. Forty-three per cent believed that interrupted sleep was implicated in their attacks. An online survey involving 407 migraineurs found that 59 per cent believed that a change in sleep pattern resulted in a migraine.

If you suspect that too little, or too much, sleep is one of your migraine triggers, or even just changes to your normal sleep routine, try to make sure you establish a regular sleep pattern and stick to it. This will mean avoiding both late nights and lie-ins as much as possible. Sleep is also one of the best ways to aid recovery during an attack. If sleep isn't possible, many sufferers find even just lying in a quiet, darkened room is helpful – in fact many sufferers find that this is the type of environment they crave during an attack. For more sleep tips, see Chapter 4 – Mind Over Migraine.

If you have to work shifts and find that this triggers attacks, try taking a melatonin supplement (see Chapter 3 – Supplementary Benefits) and using light therapy (see Useful Products) to reduce the impact on your body clock.

## 38 Cope with summer, Christmas and the working day

### Summertime blues

The summer can trigger migraines. Extremes of temperature experienced when leaving a cool, air-conditioned building to go outdoors in high temperatures can spark an attack. In warm temperatures you're likely to perspire more and therefore have a higher risk of becoming dehydrated. Bright sunlight can be a trigger for some migraineurs.

Sudden rain and thunderstorms can precipitate migraines among those who are sensitive to changes in barometric pressure. Levels of allergens, such as mould spores and pollen, are higher during the spring and summer and increased humidity following a storm can raise them further. Humid conditions also encourage dust mites – another potential allergen. Some sufferers claim their migraine attacks are due to an allergy.

Dr Mauskop, in his book *What Your Doctor May Not Tell You About Migraines*, claims that in some rare cases there is a link between allergies and migraines. He believes that the inflammation that occurs during an allergic reaction can irritate the blood vessels, including those around the brain, leading to a migraine attack. However, according to The Migraine Trust, allergies have been ruled out as the cause of migraine in most cases.

Stormy weather can also lead to higher concentrations of positive ions in the air, which some people believe may be a migraine trigger.

The heat can also reduce appetite, so there's a risk of developing low blood sugar. All of these factors can mean that the number of attacks you experience increases during the summer months.

What can you do? If you find that bright sunlight brings on a migraine, buy the best pair of sunglasses you can afford and make sure you have them with you at all times – you never know when the sun is going to shine. Wrap-around designs block out the most light, and high UV resistance and polarised lenses may also be beneficial.

Whilst there is not much you can do about the weather, you can do your best to minimise other triggers to keep attacks at bay.

- Try to wear cotton clothing and wear layers, like a cardigan or jumper, so that you can put clothes on or remove them according to the temperature.

- Even if your appetite is poor, aim to eat regular meals (small ones if that is all you can manage) with protein and wholegrains to keep blood sugar levels steady.
- Make sure you drink plenty of fluids – especially water, when the temperature rises.

## Take the headache out of Christmas

Christmas is another time when migraine sufferers may experience more attacks than usual. This is probably because you're likely to encounter more migraine triggers. The stress of last-minute Christmas shopping and preparations for Christmas Day, indulging in more alcohol than usual and the changes in routine such as late nights and lie-ins can all contribute.

Here are some tips to help take the headache out of Christmas:

- Plan ahead – don't leave your Christmas shopping and preparations until the last minute.
- Avoid money worries by drawing up a budget and sticking to it.
- Ask for help on the day.
- Avoid particular drinks – such as red wine, if you've identified them as a trigger.
- Avoid drinking alcohol on an empty stomach – eat beforehand, to slow down absorption.

- Moderate your drinking by alternating alcoholic drinks with non-alcoholic ones and prevent dehydration by drinking plenty of water before bed.
- Minimise the effects of a late night by not lying-in.

## Work it out

You may encounter several potential migraine triggers in the course of an average working day. These include work-related stress, glare from lighting and computer screens, your posture at work and even fumes from office furnishings.

### Stress less!

Work-related stress can be reduced by following many of the tips outlined in Chapter 4 – Mind over Migraine. Time management, assertiveness skills and taking regular breaks away from your desk to stretch your legs are especially important.

### Be glare aware

If you find that the flicker from your computer screen brings on migraine attacks, ensure you take regular breaks away from your desk. Use an anti-glare screen, or fit an anti-glare filter. Even just turning down the contrast could help.

Fluorescent lights also flicker and are linked to headaches. If you feel that your office lighting is a factor in your migraines, you're within your rights to ask your employer to make changes. The Workplace (Health, Safety and Welfare) Regulations stipulate that work places should have adequate and, as far as possible, natural lighting. Fluorescent lighting, dazzle and glare should be avoided and desk lights, or uplighters, should be provided. Blinds should be fitted at windows to keep out bright sunlight.

## Beat neck pain

Sitting at a desk for prolonged periods can put strain on the neck muscles and lead to neck and shoulder pain. Many migraineurs, myself included, find that neck and shoulder pain is implicated in their migraines and is often apparent before, during, or after, an attack.

Sir Robin McKenzie, the late physiotherapist who specialised in spinal problems and authored *Treat Your Own Neck*, claimed that poor sitting posture is the most common cause of neck pain and that once neck problems have developed, poor posture will exacerbate them.

To avoid tension in the neck and shoulders, watch your posture and ensure your chair and desk are the correct height for you. Your chair should be adjusted so that your feet can rest flat on the floor. Alternatively, use a footrest. Your keyboard should be at the same level as your elbows and your computer screen should be positioned so that you're looking straight ahead and not having to twist your neck or shoulders. If you are not sure whether your workspace is suited to your needs, ask your employers to check that it complies with Health and Safety Regulations.

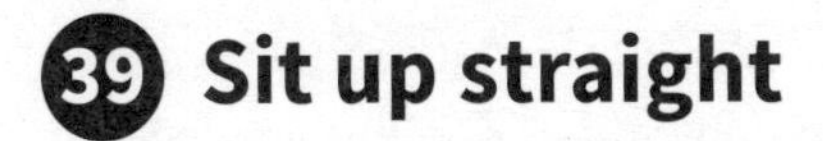

## 39 Sit up straight

According to Sir Robin, one of the main problems is how we sit. Slouching in a chair makes our head and neck protrude, which overstretches the ligaments and causes distortion of the discs and leads to pain. He recommended sitting upright, with the lower back slightly hollowed – preferably using a lumbar roll for support (see Useful Products), and keeping the upper back, neck and head straight with the chin slightly tucked in.

If you spend long periods sitting, Sir Robin also recommended practising the following exercises five or six times every hour.

### Head retraction

Head retraction involves sitting and looking straight ahead, whilst slowly pulling your head backwards as far as you can, keeping your chin tucked in. Hold for a few seconds and then relax. Repeat five or six times.

### Neck extension

For the neck extension, hold your head in the retracted position, then lift your chin up and tilt your head backwards as far as you can whilst looking up at the ceiling. Remain in this position and turn your head about 2 cm to the left and then to the right. After a few seconds return to the starting position.

Details of Sir Robin's book, *Treat Your Own Neck*, can be found in the Helpful Reading section.

**Simple neck stretch**

This exercise was recommended to me by a chiropractor. Sitting upright, slowly tilt your head towards your left shoulder, whilst dropping your right shoulder slightly. Next tilt your head to the right, dropping your left shoulder. Repeat on each side several times. To increase the stretch, place the hand from the side you are stretching towards the other side of your head and press gently.

## 40 Use the power of plants

Fumes from office equipment and soft furnishings are another possible migraine trigger. Plants make great air purifiers and are thought to reduce stress levels. Spider plants and rubber plants are fairly easy to care for.

## 41 Clean your home naturally

If you suspect that chemical-laden household cleaners are a migraine trigger for you, try using natural alternatives.

- White vinegar makes a great all-purpose cleaner. Simply dilute with an equal amount of water.
- Lemon juice contains citric acid which makes it a great natural cleaner. It has bleaching, antiseptic, antibacterial and degreasant qualities. Try cleaning the bath and wash-

basin by rubbing them with half a lemon and then rinsing with warm water.

- Olive oil is a good natural substitute for commercial furniture polish. Simply mix a cup of ordinary olive oil – it doesn't need to be extra-virgin – with the juice of one lemon and pour it into a spray bottle. To polish wooden surfaces, spray a little on to the surface and rub. The lemon juice cuts through the dirt, whilst the olive oil shines and protects the wood.
- Bicarbonate of soda is cheap and highly versatile. Mixed with water, it forms an alkaline solution that helps dissolve dirt and grease and neutralise odours. It can be used on carpets to remove stains. To clean a drain, sprinkle one cupful of bicarbonate of soda into it, then slowly pour in one cup of white vinegar. Sprinkle it on a damp cloth to clean plastic, porcelain, glass, tiles and stainless steel.
- Essential oils such as lavender, lemon or peppermint, make effective air-fresheners. Simply add a few drops to a spray bottle containing water and a little white vinegar.

Chapter 7

# Medical and Other Treatments

So you have followed the advice in this book. You have identified your migraine triggers and are doing your best to avoid them. Maybe you have changed your eating habits and started taking one or two supplements. However, unless you are very lucky, you are still likely to suffer from a migraine attack from time to time. This is when it is important to know what medications are available that can help you during an attack. These are known as acute treatments. If you are really unlucky and find you still have frequent attacks, you probably need to consider taking a preventative (prophylactic) drug.

You may find over-the-counter treatments effective – in this chapter you'll find an overview of the medications currently available without prescription. However, if you try a few of these without success, it is important that you seek help from your GP, as they will be able to prescribe stronger painkillers or other acute or preventative medications.

Dr Peter Goadsby, who works with The Migraine Trust and is a professor of neurology at the Institute of Neurology at University College, London, is keen on sufferers helping themselves by identifying triggers and adapting their lifestyles to reduce attacks. However, he wants migraineurs and GPs to become more aware of what can be done about migraine. He believes that about 50 per cent of migraineurs fail to receive suitable medication to prevent or treat their condition, either because they suffer in silence, or because their GP fails to accurately diagnose their condition or prescribe the correct treatment. According to Professor Goadsby, 'every migraineur has an individual pattern' and therefore it is 'not a good idea just to blanket prescribe anti-migraine drugs.' He advises that GPs need to be aware of the type of migraine a patient is suffering from, as well as the frequency of attacks. He points out that someone who suffers from a two-hour migraine once a fortnight may not want to take a daily migraine preventative, whereas someone suffering ten a month might.

When you visit your GP it is important to provide detailed information about your attacks to ensure you receive the correct diagnosis and medication if you need it. You'll find more advice about how to prepare for a doctor's appointment in the Introduction.

This chapter looks at the treatments currently available, as well as new ones in the developmental stage and when and how these may be of benefit. We also look at a couple of practical self-help treatments and end with five top tips to beat a migraine attack.

# 42 Learn about medications for migraine

It is strongly recommended that you take painkillers as soon as an attack starts, because once a migraine attack is underway, your body's systems, including digestion, tend to slow down so drugs are less readily absorbed. Even basic painkillers such as aspirin and ibuprofen can be enough to abort an attack when taken soon enough. If you do not take medication early on, it is unlikely that you will benefit and the attack will be more severe and last longer. The exception to this is a group of drugs known as triptans, which are more effective when taken once the headache has begun (see below). Soluble tablets are absorbed more quickly than non-soluble ones. If you feel nauseous, tablets that fizz may be easier to keep down. Alternatively, try taking ordinary tablets with sparkling water or a fizzy drink.

## Medication to go!

As migraines can often develop unexpectedly, it is important to get into the habit of carrying a dose of your medication around with you so that you can always catch it early, wherever you are. Carrying a snack such as a muesli bar, plain digestive biscuits with a small bottle of water, or fruit juice means you will not have to take your medication on an empty stomach.

## Over-the-counter treatments

For some sufferers, over-the-counter painkillers are effective if taken early enough. Medications that you can buy without a prescription to treat headaches will contain one or more of these drugs:

**Antihistamines** – can help to prevent nausea, but may also have a sedative effect.

**Aspirin** – a non-steroidal anti-inflammatory drug (NSAID) that relieves mild to moderate pain and reduces inflammation and a high body temperature. Aspirin can damage the lining of your stomach, so avoid taking it if you have a stomach ulcer. It is also not suitable for asthma sufferers.

**Caffeine** – can improve the absorption of your painkiller. Usually only a small amount is included, but tablets containing caffeine are best avoided near bedtime as caffeine is a stimulant that may cause wakefulness. You could get the same effect by taking an ordinary painkiller with a cup of coffee or a glass of cola.

**Codeine** – is one of the opiate family of drugs, which includes morphine and heroin, hence it's only allowed in small quantities in over-the-counter medications. Even small amounts can cause constipation, it can be addictive and, if taken often, can cause rebound headaches. It may also cause dizziness and sedation. It enhances the effects of other painkillers.

**Ibuprofen** – another non-steroidal anti-inflammatory drug (NSAID) that relieves pain and reduces inflammation. It is less likely to irritate the stomach, but it's not recommended for anyone with high blood pressure, kidney problems, asthma or a stomach ulcer.

**Paracetamol** – also relieves pain and reduces fever. Paracetamol shouldn't cause any side effects when the recommended dose is taken, however, it is toxic to the liver, so overdosing is potentially very dangerous. This drug shouldn't be taken by anyone with kidney or liver problems.

Proprietary preparations containing these drugs include Migraleve, Midrid, Propain and Syndol – see the Useful Products section for more information.

## Anti-nausea and anti-vomiting treatments (anti-emetics)

If you suffer from severe nausea and vomiting during an attack, it may be worth taking an over-the-counter anti-emetic, along with a painkiller. This could help to relieve the nausea as well as improve your absorption of the painkiller. Over-the-counter anti-emetic drugs include:

**Buccastem M** – contains prochlorperazine – a type of medicine called a phenothiazine – which, in low doses can help to relieve nausea and vomiting associated with migraines. The prochlorperazine works by blocking the receptors for the brain chemical dopamine in an area of the brain that controls nausea and vomiting.

**Gaviscon** – is a medication for heartburn and indigestion which some sufferers find helps when taken with painkillers. For further information see the Useful Products section.

**Migraleve** – combines codeine, paracetamol and an anti-emetic. Note: Taking codeine regularly for more than three days can cause addiction and withdrawal symptoms when stopped. You can find further information about this medication in the Useful Products section.

**Motilium** – contains domperidone, which helps the digestive system to return to normal. It's thought to work by affecting areas of the brain that are linked to nausea and vomiting. Domperidone is also available on prescription, in tablet or suppository form.

## Prescription medications

If over-the-counter medications prove ineffective, your GP can prescribe more powerful medications, such as:

**Stronger NSAIDS (non-steroidal anti-inflammatory drugs)** – including diclofenac, naproxen and tolfenamic acid.

**Anti-emetics** – such as metoclopramide.

**Anti-emetics and painkillers combined** – such as Migramax, Domperamol and Paramax.

## Triptans

If painkillers or anti-inflammatories don't help during an attack, it may be worth trying one of the triptans. There are several types, including naratriptan, sumatriptan, almotriptan, eletriptan, frovatriptan, rizatriptan, and zolmitriptan – each one has a different brand name. Triptans are not painkillers. Also known as serotonin (5HT) agonists, they work by balancing the levels of serotonin in the brain, which enables the swollen blood vessels to return to their normal size and calms down the sensory nerves. They are generally only available on prescription, except for one product – Imigran Recovery – an over-the-counter medication that contains sumatriptan. You will first need to complete a questionnaire to determine your suitability for the treatment. This is available in pharmacies and on the product website. For more information about Imigran Recovery, see the Useful Products section. Imigran is also available as an injection and a nasal spray on prescription

Zolmitriptan is available as a nasal spray called Zomig, it is sprayed into one nostril to relieve a migraine attack. It is absorbed into the bloodstream through blood vessels in the nose and starts to work within around 15 minutes. This means it is likely to be absorbed more quickly and easily than oral (tablet) forms, because most sufferers find their digestive processes slow down during an attack. It is also useful for people who experience nausea or vomiting during migraines and therefore find it difficult to keep tablets down, though some people may find the spray leaves a taste in the mouth that makes the nausea worse.

Rizatriptan and zolmitriptan are also available in formulations that dissolve in the mouth, which is also useful if swallowing proves difficult and it means they enter into the bloodstream and start working quicker than tablets. At the time of writing, a triptan patch aimed at those who have problems taking both tablets and sprays is undergoing clinical trials in the US.

Unlike painkillers, triptans shouldn't be taken too early; rather than taking them at the first sign of an attack, for example during the aura stage, take them when the headache has begun, as research has shown they are more effective at this stage.

Generally, if the first dose doesn't work, you are advised not to take another one as this is also likely to be ineffective. The exception is zolmitriptan, if the first dose doesn't work, a second can be tried. Usually no more than two doses can be taken in 24 hours – though this can vary.

Triptans can be taken alongside standard painkillers and anti-emetics if they are needed. Research suggests that taking a triptan with an NSAID is more effective than combining it with paracetamol. Your GP may prescribe a larger dose if necessary. If one triptan doesn't work, it may be worth trying another one. It's recommended that you try one for at least two or three attacks before making any judgement as, for various reasons, it may not be effective every time. See your GP about trying another type, if the first one doesn't seem to help.

Triptans are safer than ergotamine, as they only constrict the swollen blood vessels, rather than blood vessels all over the body. However, there are a number of possible side effects, so always make sure you read the patient information leaflet carefully.

Common side effects include drowsiness, feeling sick (nausea), dizziness and dry mouth. Some people experience feelings of warmth, tingling, tightness, heaviness or pressure in the face or limbs or sometimes in the chest, These usually develop within half an hour and shouldn't last long. However, if you develop intense sensations or chest pain, have an allergic reaction, i.e. wheezing, swelling, breathlessness or collapse, or a fit, you should stop taking the medication and seek immediate medical attention.

Another problem is that the migraine can return later on. A further dose can be taken but sometimes the migraine can reappear. Also be aware that overuse of triptans can make migraines worse and more frequent, so avoid taking them more than twice a week on a regular basis.

**Note**

Don't take triptans if you suffer from heart disease, stroke, high blood pressure, epilepsy, circulation problems, or if you suffer from any of the more rare forms of migraines. Don't take sumatriptan (Imigran) or naratriptan (Naramig), if you are allergic to sulphonamide antibiotics.

**Painkiller/triptan overuse**

Research has shown that overuse of painkillers such as paracetamol, aspirin or triptans can lead to 'rebound' headaches. It seems that taking painkillers regularly leads to the body stopping the production of its own painkilling systems, resulting in more headaches or migraines. Another possibility is that your body becomes used to the painkillers or triptan; if you don't take another dose within a day or so of the last one you develop a withdrawal (rebound) headache. Only strong painkillers carry a warning that overuse can worsen headaches – aspirin, paracetamol and ibuprofen do not.

## Preventative (prophylactic) treatments

If you regularly experience more than two attacks per month that disrupt your everyday life, or suffer from especially severe or prolonged attacks, your GP may recommend a course of preventative drugs. Antihypertensives (drugs that lower blood pressure) anti-epileptic, antihistamine and anti-depressant drugs have been found to be effective and include:

### Propranolol

Propranolol is a beta blocker used to treat various conditions, including high blood pressure and cardiovascular disease. It helps to relax the blood vessels and can be effective in the prevention of migraine attacks. However, potential side effects include muscle fatigue, sleep disturbance, dizziness, sedation, cold extremities (fingers and toes), pins and needles and numbness.

### Topiramate (Topamax)

Topiramate is an anti-epilepsy drug that can now be prescribed to migraineurs after trials showed it may help to reduce the frequency of attacks by up to half. Taken daily as a preventative, the drug is an anti-convulsant that also has an effect on calcium levels in the body – low levels are thought to be a possible migraine trigger. Levels of the drug build up in the system and reduce the chance of an attack. It's thought that topiramate works well for migraines because there seems to be a link between the chemical pathways in the brain involved in epilepsy and those implicated in migraines.

Common side effects of topiramate include tingling in arms and legs, loss of appetite, nausea, weight loss, taste change, diarrhoea, nervousness, speech and memory problems, stomach pain, tiredness, fever and eye problems. According to my consultant and GP, some people are unable to tolerate the side effects of this drug, while others claim it has completely transformed their lives.

### Gabapentin

If propranolol or topiramate prove unsuitable or ineffective, your GP may prescribe gabapentin, another anti-epileptic drug.

Most people can take gabapentin, but it should be used with caution in people with kidney problems and those aged over 65 years.

Side effects of gabapentin can include dizziness, drowsiness, increased appetite, weight gain and suicidal thoughts.

### Other drugs

If propranolol, topirimate or gabapentin prove unsuitable or ineffective, your GP may prescribe another preventative drug, such as amitriptyline, sodium valproate or pizotifen. However, evidence of how effective they are is limited.

### Amitriptyline

Amitriptyline is an antidepressant that can be useful in preventing migraines that appear to be linked to depression. It is also thought to have an anti-migraine action that is separate from its antidepressant properties. A low dose is given to start with, which is then increased, if necessary. Common side effects include a dry mouth, drowsiness, blurred vision, and nausea and digestive problems.

### Sodium valproate

Sodium valproate is another anti-epileptic drug that can help prevent migraines in some people. Exactly how it works is unknown, but the drug is thought to slow down brain activity. Possible side effects of sodium valproate include nausea, digestive problems and stomach pain, weight gain and temporary hair loss. Rare side effects include rashes and impaired platelet and liver function.

### Pizotifen

The antihistamine known as pizotifen (Sanomigran) is also sometimes used as a migraine preventative. It affects serotonin levels and acts as an antidepressant. But it can cause sleepiness and increased appetite, leading to weight gain, so it's not usually prescribed for adults by migraine specialists.

# 43 Discover other treatments

New and innovative treatments for preventing migraines are being researched and tested all the time. The following are some of the alternative treatments used to treat migraines.

## Acupuncture

Traditional acupuncture is a treatment stemming from ancient Chinese medicine, in which ultra-fine sterile needles are inserted at specific points in the body for therapeutic or preventative purposes. It is based on the belief that pain and illness are caused by the disruption of the flow of vital energy or qi in the body; the insertion of needles is thought to restore the flow of qi to recover balance and trigger the body's natural healing response. Traditional acupuncture is performed by more than a million acupuncturists worldwide. The British Acupuncture Council is the leading self-regulatory body for the practice of traditional acupuncture in the UK.

Medical acupuncture used in Western medicine, usually by physiotherapists, doctors and nurses, is an adaptation of traditional acupuncture; sometimes known as 'dry needling'. Its use is based on scientific evidence that it stimulates nerves under the skin and in the muscle tissue, which encourages the body to release pain-relieving substances, such as endorphins. Medical acupuncture is overseen by the British Medical Acupuncture Society (BMAS) and the Acupuncture Association of Chartered Physiotherapists (AACP).

According to the British Acupuncture Council there is evidence that acupuncture also helps migraine by:

- Changing the brain's processing of pain.
- Reducing inflammation.
- Balancing blood flow in and around the brain.
- Balancing serotonin levels.
- Reducing levels of calcitonin gene-related peptide (CGRP) and substance P (brain chemicals involved in migraine).
- Reducing cortical spreading depression (an electrical brain wave linked to blood flow changes in brain).

Other theories suggest that acupuncture has a pain de-sensitising effect and raises the migaine threshold so that more triggers are needed to start an attack.

Even if you dislike needles, you shouldn't have a problem with acupuncture, as the needles are very fine. At the time of writing I've been having regular treatments for over a year and find that I don't feel most of the needles going in – though I might feel slight discomfort at one or two sites; in general, I find the treatments quite relaxing.

In 2012, NICE recommended a course of ten acupuncture treatments for migraine prevention, based on evidence that it is as effective as preventative medications. These will usually be offerered at a specialist migraine clinic, although some GP practices offer integrated healthcare that includes acupuncture – unfortunately this is not yet commonplace. One point to be aware of is that your migraines may return once the treatments cease.

If this happens, you may want to continue having treatments with a private acupuncturist. Always choose an acupuncturist who is registered with the British Acupuncture Council (see Directory). You may need frequent treatments at the beginning, but eventually these should reduce to anything from one every three weeks to one every six months, depending on the severity of your migraines and your response to acupuncture.

## Botox injections

In 2012, The National Institute for Health and Care Excellence (NICE) recommended botulinum toxin type A to be administered by a headache specialist to prevent chronic migraine in sufferers who hadn't responded to at least three preventative medications.

Botulinum toxin type A is a type of nerve toxin that paralyses muscles. It is not exactly clear why this treatment can be effective for migraine.

The treatment should be given by injection to between 31 and 39 sites around the head and back of the neck every 12 weeks. While the treatment is recommended by NICE, the ease of access to it will depend on whether funding is available via your local Clinical Commissioning Group (CCG.)

## Calcitonin gene-related peptide (CGRP) antagonists

This medication blocks the release of CGRP in the brain during an attack. Calcitonin gene-related peptide is a brain chemical that causes blood vessels in the brain to dilate and is thought to be implicated in migraine. In the UK, the generic CGRP (flunarizine) isn't widely available and only tends to be prescribed by a migraine specialist.

## Greater occipital nerve block

The greater occipital nerve block is a fairly common procedure for the treatment of migraine in people who fail to respond to medications, or who suffer bad side effects from them. It involves injecting a local anaesthetic, usually combined with a steroid, into the greater occipital nerve (GON) at the back of the head to block pain. This area of the brain processes vision, including colour recognition, spatial awareness and word recognition. Most migraineurs experience tenderness in the sub-occipital area.

The practitioner finds the GON by finding the area at the back of the head where the patient feels the most pain or tenderness. The injection, which is done with a small, very thin needle, takes a few minutes and is uncomfortable rather than painful. Some people notice a warm feeling at the back of their heads after the treatment, but this doesn't last for long. The anaesthetic begins to take effect after a few minutes and the steroid in the injection should start to work between one to seven days later. The pain-relieving effects can last anything from several days to a few months and can vary from one person to another.

This is a relatively safe procedure that only takes a few minutes to administer. It's usually well tolerated and side effects like numbness or pain at the back of the head should disappear within a few hours. People who have the treatment are advised to avoid driving for a few hours but can normally return to work within 24 hours.

## Transcranial magnetic stimulation

NICE approved the use of a treatment called transcranial magnetic stimulation (TMS) for the prevention and treatment of migraines in 2014.

TMS involves holding a small electrical device to your head that sends out magnetic pulses. It is thought that TMS treats migraines by 'short-circuiting' their development. It can be used alone or combined with medications mentioned above, without interfering with them.

However, TMS isn't a cure for migraines and it doesn't work for everybody. There isn't strong evidence of its effectiveness and it only works for people who suffer from migraine with aura.

Also, there isn't much evidence about the potential long-term effects of the treatment, although so far trials have reported only mild, temporary side effects, including slight dizziness and drowsiness, irritability and muscle tremor. Because of the uncertainty about the potential long-term side effects, NICE recommends that TMS should only be provided by headache professionals at specialist centres where patients' experiences of the treatment will be recorded.

## 44 Try self-help treatments

**Blood flow reduction**

It is claimed that reducing the flow of blood to swollen blood vessels in the head can help to relieve migraines. Tie a bandage around your forehead and tighten it until you can feel the pressure right around your head.

**Blow hot – or cold!**

Some people find an ice pack (or a towel wrung out in icy cold water) applied to the back of the neck or the temples relieves migraine pain. The cool temperature will help to constrict the blood vessels and reduce the flow of blood to the brain.

Others find that heat helps – perhaps in the form of a hot wheat pillow, a towel wrung out in hot water or even soaking in a hot bath. Heat applied to the forehead or nape of the neck will help to dilate the blood vessels and increase the blood flow to the brain. Try both to find out which one, if any, helps you – obviously it will depend on whether the pain is due to constricted or swollen blood vessels around the brain. You can buy wheat pillows that you simply heat up in the microwave. Some contain lavender which can help to ease headaches. You can also buy 'cool caps' such as the Migra-Cap – for more information see the Useful Products section.

## Five top tips to beat migraines

When a migraine strikes it is important to act quickly to minimise the effects. Also, many people find themselves totally incapacitated once the attack is under way, so it makes sense to start treating yourself whilst you still feel able to do so. Following these tips should help you to abort an attack as quickly as possible.

**Medicate** – take your preferred painkillers at the first signs of an attack. Take triptans at the start of the headache.

**Eat** – if you feel you can eat, go for a light snack of wholegrain and protein, for example a sandwich with tuna, turkey or cheese on wholemeal bread, or even plain biscuits, such as digestives. If low blood sugar has contributed to the attack, this may help to shorten it.

**Drink** – coffee or cola help to boost the efficiency of painkillers. Drink a glass or two of water in case dehydration has precipitated an attack.

**Apply heat or cold** – whichever works for you – to your forehead and the nape of your neck if the muscles are tense there.

**Sleep** – or just rest in a quiet, darkened room. Wear an eye mask if it helps (see Useful Products).

There will probably be occasions when a migraine strikes and you are not able to, or do not want to, stop what you are doing. If you follow the first three tips: medicate, eat and drink, you may be able to 'soldier on'. If you can fit in half an hour's rest as well, so much the better. Be warned, though: I have found that if I do not 'give in' to a migraine and rest for at least a couple of hours early on in the attack, it can take longer to recover and return to normal.

Chapter 8

# DIY Complementary Therapies

This chapter gives you an overview and evaluation of complementary therapies – from acupressure to yoga – that may improve your well-being and reduce the frequency or duration of migraine attacks. It also offers techniques and treatments you can try for yourself.

## 45 Apply acupressure

Acupressure is part of traditional Chinese medicine and is often described as 'acupuncture without needles'. Like acupuncture, it's based on the idea that life energy, or qi, flows through channels in the body known as meridians. An even passage of qi throughout the body is viewed as essential to good health. Disruption of the flow of qi in a meridian can lead to illness at any point within it. The flow of qi can be affected by various factors including stress, emotional distress, diet and environment. Qi is the most concentrated at points along the meridians known as acupoints. There's scientific evidence that stimulating particular acupoints can relieve both pain and nausea.

**Meeting of the valleys**

This is an acupoint, also known as Hoku, positioned in the web between the thumb and forefinger of both hands. Apply firm pressure downwards, towards the forefinger, to one hand and then the other, to relieve migraine pain and help ease the digestive problems often associated with an attack. You can buy a wrist strap that applies constant pressure to this acupoint (see Useful Products for more details).

**Inner gate**

Also known as the Nei Kuan, this is an acupoint positioned on the forearm, about 5 cm down from the first wrist crease and in line with the ring finger. Apply pressure here to relieve the nausea associated with migraines. You can also buy an acupressure band for your wrist, that exerts pressure on this area and thus relieves nausea. See the Useful Products section for more details.

**Neck tension relief**

Migraines are often linked to a tense, aching neck and shoulders. The trapezius muscle runs along from the base of the neck to the shoulder and is an acupoint which, if stimulated, can help to relieve tension and ease headache pain. Press firmly along the muscle, focusing on any area that is particularly tender.

# 46 Ease pain with essential oils

Essential oils are extracted from the roots, stalks, leaves and flowers of plants.

Aromatherapy is based on the idea that scents released from essential oils affect the hypothalamus, the part of the brain which controls the glands and hormonal system, thus influencing mood and lowering stress levels. As stress is a major migraine trigger, anything that can relieve stress has the potential to reduce the frequency of attacks. Because essential oils are concentrated, some may sting when applied directly to the skin. The general recommendation is to add one or two drops to one teaspoon of a carrier oil, such as olive, sunflower, almond, or wheatgerm. Good quality culinary versions will do.

## Lavender compress

Some oils, such as lavender, have calming and pain-relieving properties. Some migraineurs gain relief during an attack by gently massaging lavender oil into the temples, or by placing a few drops just inside the nostrils. Alternatively, if you find heat helps to ease the pain, place a warm compress sprinkled with lavender oil, or a hot wheat pillow containing lavender, either on your forehead, or on the back of your neck – especially if there is pain and tension there. Lavender can be used neat, but this can cause a skin reaction. If you are affected, dilute two drops in one teaspoon of carrier oil before applying it to the skin.

### Pep up with peppermint

Evidence suggests that peppermint oil can relieve the pain and nausea of a migraine attack. The active ingredient, menthol, is the main ingredient of a range of headache medications called 4Head – see the Useful Products section. It is thought to ease pain by cooling and numbing the area to which it is applied. It also boosts blood flow to the area and reduces substance P, a brain chemical involved in pain transmission. Add a few drops to hot or cold water and soak a small towel or facecloth. Wring out the excess moisture and use as a compress on the forehead or neck. Dilute two drops in a carrier oil and massage into your stomach. If you're out and about, sprinkle a few drops of peppermint oil onto a handkerchief and inhale, or put just one drop on your index fingertip and massage into your forehead and the nape of your neck.

Patricia Davis, author of the *Aromatherapy A–Z*, suggests that a combination of peppermint and lavender oils may be even more effective in relieving symptoms.

**Note**

Drinking peppermint tea can also ease nausea and help clear the head. Remember, however, that peppermint is a stimulant, so avoid using it close to bedtime.

## Rosemary relief

Both the medical herbalist Andrew Chevallier and the Herb Society, recommend rosemary for migraines. Chevallier points to its anti-inflammatory and circulation-boosting properties. The Herb Society describes it as a tonic for depression, anxiety and nervous migraines. Dilute it first and then massage it into your forehead and the back of your neck or, alternatively, place a couple of drops on a handkerchief and inhale.

## Herbal healing

Herbalists commonly prescribe the following herbs to help relieve migraines:

**German camomile** – to relieve pain and aid relaxation.

**Skullcap** – to relieve tension – it is also antispasmodic.

**Valerian** – for its antispasmodic, calming and sedative effects.

**Lemon balm** – to soothe and calm an overactive mind.

**Betony** – is thought to stimulate the circulation and aid relaxation.

Try taking these herbs as an infusion (tea). Make your own, using 30 g (2 tbsp) of fresh herbs or 10 g (2 tsp) of dried herbs. Pour boiling water over the herb, cover and leave to stand for about ten minutes. Strain and add honey to taste. Drink whilst hot. There are also ready-made herbal teas containing single, or combined, herbs that are available in health stores.

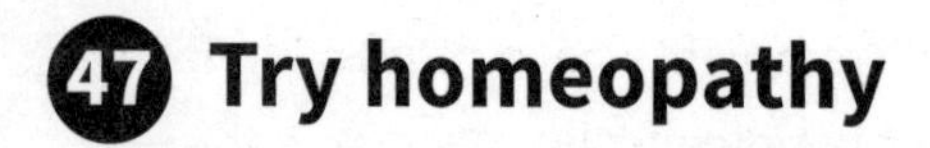

# 47 Try homeopathy

Homeopathy means 'same suffering' and is based on the belief that 'like cures like': substances that can cause symptoms in a well person, can treat the same symptoms in an ill person. Symptoms such as inflammation or fever are seen as a sign that the body is attempting to heal itself. Homeopathic remedies are designed to stimulate this self-healing process and they are thought to work in a similar way to vaccines.

The substances used in homeopathic remedies are derived from plant, animal and mineral sources. These substances are used to produce a tincture that is then diluted many times. Homeopaths claim that the more diluted a remedy is, the higher its potency and the lower its potential side effects. This idea is based on the 'memory of water' theory which claims that though molecules from substances have been diluted away, they have left behind an electromagnetic 'footprint' – like a recording on an audiotape – which exerts an effect on the body.

These ideas are controversial, with many GPs remaining sceptical. Evidence to support homeopathy exists, but much of it is deemed inconclusive. In 2004 a review of the evidence for the homeopathic treatment of headaches (including migraines) concluded that overall homeopathy was safe and might benefit headache sufferers, but there was a lack of convincing evidence that it was more effective than a placebo. The review also criticised the design of the studies so far and recommended further research. However, some migraine sufferers claim to have been helped by homeopathy, so it may be worth trying, especially if conventional treatments have proved ineffective, or have caused unacceptable side effects.

There are two main types of remedy: whole person based and symptom based. A homeopath would prescribe a remedy based on your personality, as well as the symptoms you experience. Homeopaths view migraines as a disease of the nervous system and prescribed remedies seek to treat the symptoms by calming the mind, encouraging the healing process and addressing an individual's particular symptoms.

The easiest way to treat yourself is to select the remedy that most closely matches your individual symptoms. Some of the remedies commonly prescribed for migraines and the symptoms for which they're claimed to be beneficial are:

**Arnica** – recommended for headaches arising from head trauma or injury.

**Belladonna** – for throbbing, pounding headaches with sensitivity to light and sound.

**Ignatia** – headaches related to grief or depression.

**Ipecac** – for pain that affects the whole head (including the face) along with nausea and vomiting.

**Iris** – for intense migraines, especially those with aura or other visual disturbance, and vomiting.

**Lachesis** – for excruciating pain, especially on the left side of the head.

**Lycopodium** – for pain that is worse on the right side and increases when trying to concentrate.

**Natrum mur** – for a throbbing, blinding headache, accompanied by a congested feeling. Also where an attack is preceded by numbness and tingling in the lips, tongue and nose.

**Nux vomica** – for migraines linked to food triggers or alcohol.

**Petroleum** – for a severe headache where there's a feeling of heaviness at the back of the head and the scalp is sensitive both to the cold and to touch.

**Pulsatilla** – for headache that's worse at night or during a period. The head feels as though it is about to burst and the sufferer may be tearful.

**Silicea** – for migraines triggered by hormones, exertion or orgasm.

**Spigelia** – for sharp, painful, throbbing headaches where stooping makes pain worse.

**Sanguinaria** – for pain on the right side of the head, extending down into the right shoulder, along with sensitivity to light and sounds.

**Note**

Practitioners caution people that homeopathy is not a 'quick fix' – the remedies may take a while to take effect. Homeopathic remedies are generally considered safe and don't have any known side effects, though sometimes a temporary worsening of symptoms, known as 'aggravation' may take place. This is seen as a good sign, as it suggests that the remedy is encouraging the healing process. If this happens, stop taking the remedy and wait for your symptoms to improve. If there is steady improvement, do not restart the remedy. If the improvement stops, resume taking the remedy.

## 48 Use the power of touch

Massage is an ancient and effective means of reducing stress, making it a useful tool for the prevention of migraines. The 'Father of Medicine', Greek philosopher Hippocrates, recognised the power of massage, claiming it 'can loosen a joint that is too rigid'. Daily stresses can make us tense and lead to pain and stiffness. Muscle tension in the neck and shoulders can trigger a migraine. Massage uses the power of touch to ease away tensions, aches and pains, whilst boosting circulation, digestion and immunity. Studies suggest it works by stimulating the release of endorphins – the body's own painkillers – and serotonin, a brain chemical linked to relaxation. It also decreases the level of stress hormones in the blood.

Mix your own massage oil by adding a few drops of your favourite aromatherapy oil to a carrier oil. Lavender and camomile are particularly relaxing. To enjoy the benefits of massage at home, you and a partner can take turns to massage each other's back, neck and shoulders, using these basic techniques:

**Stroking/effleurage** – glide both hands over the skin in slow, rhythmic fanning or circular motions.

**Kneading** – using alternate hands, squeeze and release flesh between fingers and thumbs.

**Friction** –using your thumbs, apply even pressure to static points on each side of the spine, or make small circles.

**Hacking** – using the sides of your hands alternately, deliver short, sharp taps all over.

Playing relaxing music at the same time can enhance relaxation. It's not just the receiver who gains from massage – apparently the giver also benefits from improved mood and higher self-esteem. Gently massaging your temples may also help to ease pain and tension during an attack.

## 49 Relax with reflexology

Reflexology is based on the idea that points on the feet, hands and face, known as reflexes, correspond to parts of the body, glands and organs. It is claimed that stimulating these reflexes, using the fingers and thumbs, brings about physiological changes, which encourage self-healing. It is thought that this is possible because energy flows through the body via ten zones, which run vertically from each foot to the head, and from the hands up to the neck and shoulders. Practitioners believe that imbalances in the body result in granular deposits in the relevant reflex, leading to tenderness. Corns, bunions and even hard skin are thought to indicate problems in the parts of the body to which their position relates.

In 1999, a Danish study of 220 people who experienced regular migraines, or tension headaches, claimed that reflexology reduced the severity of symptoms in 61 per cent of cases and completely cured symptoms in another 16 per cent. Whilst medical opinion is divided, evidence suggests that foot and hand massage can reduce stress, and as such may well benefit migraine sufferers.

## Simple hand reflexology

If you want to self-treat, it is easier and more convenient to practice on your hands rather than your feet. The movements outlined below will contact the reflexes linked to the digestive system, liver and kidneys, and are recommended by practitioners for the relief of migraines.

Warm up each hand by kneading each palm with the fist of your other hand.

Using the right thumb on the left palm, start about a quarter of the way up the inner edge, creep forward slowly towards the left thumb, pressing down firmly. Continue working across the palm from left to right, working your way up to about 2 cm below the base of the fingers. Repeat on the right hand using the left thumb.

## Neck and shoulder treatment

Many migraine sufferers experience neck and shoulder pain before or during an attack. The following techniques are designed to work on these areas.

**To relieve neck pain** – use your right thumb to creep around the base of your left thumb, applying firm pressure. Repeat several times.

**To relieve shoulder pain** – using the right thumb, creep up the middle of the little finger on your left hand, starting from the base and finishing at the tip. Repeat several times and then perform the same movements on your right hand, using your left thumb.

# 50 Try yoga

The BMJ Best Treatments website (run by the British Medical Association's publishing division, the British Medical Journal Publishing Group) recommends yoga for treatment of migraines. The word 'yoga' comes from the Sanskrit word yuj, meaning union. Yogic postures and breathing exercises are designed to unite the body, mind and soul. It is a gentle form of exercise that strengthens the body and increases flexibility, as well as inducing calm, relieving stress and easing aches and pains.

## Useful postures

Inverted postures, like the shoulder stand, boost circulation and blood flow to the upper body. The plough relieves stiffness in the neck and shoulders. The cobra releases tension and stiffness in the neck and back muscles.

## Yogic breathing

Yogic breathing, or Pranayama, revitalises the whole body, balances the emotions and clears the mind. Pranayama is best performed sitting down, holding the spine, neck and head in a straight line. This promotes the flow of Prana (life energy) and allows the lungs to expand fully.

1. Sit cross-legged on a yoga block or cushion to relieve tension in the lower back and knees. Put one hand on your ribcage and the other on your tummy. Your back should be straight with your chin parallel to the floor and your shoulders relaxed.
2. Inhale slowly and deeply through your nose with your mouth closed, allowing your stomach to expand first, then your ribcage and then your whole chest area.
3. Exhale slowly through your nostrils, allowing the air to leave your lower lungs first, then the ribcage area and finally the chest.

**Learn yoga**

The best way to learn yoga is to attend classes run by a qualified teacher. To find one near you, go to the British Wheel of Yoga's website – www.bwy.org.uk. Or, if you would prefer to teach yourself at home, visit www.abc-of-yoga.com – a site that shows you how to do the various postures; www.yoga-abode.com and www.yogaatwork.co.uk, also offer information, guidance and yoga products.

# Jargon Buster

A lot of books about migraines, including this one, use terms whose meaning you may be unsure of. Listed here are the meanings of some words and phrases that might be used when describing the diagnosis, treatment and prevention of migraines.

**Acute** – the rapid onset of a condition, when symptoms are severe, such as migraines. An acute treatment is used to treat an attack once it's under way, rather than to prevent it.

**Agonist** – a drug that binds to receptor cells and produces an action, often mimicking the action of a natural substance. For example, 5HT agonists mimic the action of the brain chemical serotonin.

**Anti-inflammatory** – drug, or other substance, that counteracts inflammation.

**Aura** – a visual disturbance that precedes a migraine attack in some sufferers.

**Carcinogenic** – a substance thought to cause cancer.

**Chronic** – persisting for a long time and, in the case of migraines, constantly recurring.

**Double-blind study** – a study design in which there are two groups of participants and one is given a placebo and the other a treatment. Neither group is aware of what they have been given, so as not to affect the result.

**Episodic** – something that happens intermittently, as in migraines.

**Metabolism** – the breaking down of substances for use in the body.

**Migraineur** – a person who suffers from migraines.

**Neurological** – relating to brain function. Migraine is classified as a neurological condition.

**Premonitory symptoms** – see prodromal phase/symptoms.

**Prodromal phase/symptoms** – the first phase of a migraine – usually the period of up to 24 hours before an attack. Symptoms sufferers may experience include mood changes, food cravings, tiredness, irritability or neck pain. Also known as premonitory symptoms.

**Prophylactic** – prevents illness.

**Rebound** – a term used to describe a migraine that occurs as a result of overuse of medication taken to treat the condition, either whilst you're still taking it or afterwards as a result of its withdrawal.

**Relapse** – this is the more recent term with the same meaning as 'rebound'.

**Uncontrolled study** – a study where there is no control (comparison) group. The results are usually deemed less reliable than those from controlled studies.

# Helpful Reading

Mole, Peter, *Acupuncture for Body, Mind and Spirit* (2007, Spring Hill)
A great introduction to acupuncture. This book covers the history of acupuncture and the philosophical basis of Chinese medicine, as well as how acupuncture is used and what to expect during a treatment.

McKenzie, Robin, *Treat Your Own Neck* (2006, Spinal Publications New Zealand Ltd)
This book is well worth reading if you suffer from neck and shoulder problems and feel they might be implicated in your migraine attacks. It contains lots of helpful advice on how to avoid neck pain by improving your posture and how to treat it through a series of exercises designed to restore mobility and relieve pain.

Sacks, Oliver, *Migraine* (1995, Picador)
Offers a comprehensive and in-depth guide to migraine, its various causes, preventative tactics and treatments. I especially like the chapter on psychological approaches to migraines.

# Useful Products

In this section there is a list of products and suppliers of products that may help to reduce the frequency or severity of migraine attacks. The author doesn't endorse or recommend any particular product and this list is by no means exhaustive – there is a vast range of items available that may help with the prevention and treatment of migraine.

**4Head Stick**

A twist-up stick containing levomenthol, a peppermint extract that has a cooling and painkilling effect when applied to the forehead. It is thought to work by relaxing the blood vessels. Available in supermarkets and pharmacies nationwide.

Website: www.4headaches.co.uk

**4Head QuickStrip**

A hydro-gel patch for use with or without painkillers or other medications that has a cooling and pain-relieving effect and helps relax tense head and neck muscles. Available in supermarkets and pharmacies nationwide.

Website: www.4headaches.co.uk

**Anatomicals Headache Relief Balm**

Aromatherapy balm containing peppermint, lavender, eucalyptus, mandarin and sandalwood oils to help relieve pain, and to calm and relax. Comes in a handy little tin that's easy to carry around with you.

Website: www.anatomicals.com.mt

**Anti-Headache Acupressure Band**

A specially designed wrist strap with an inbuilt pressure button that applies constant gentle pressure to the Hoku (L14) acupoint. Available on Amazon.

Website: www.amazon.co.uk

**Eurovital Melatonin**

Capsules containing 3 mg of melatonin.

Website: www.biovea.net/UK

**Gaviscon**

A range of over-the-counter antacids for the relief of heartburn and indigestion. Some migraine sufferers find that they help with the digestive symptoms that accompany an attack. Available at pharmacies nationwide.

Website: www.gaviscon.co.uk

**Gelstat Migraine**

An over-the-counter homeopathic gel that contains feverfew and ginger. The product is poured under the tongue; the manufacturers claim that this allows the medication to be absorbed more quickly.

Website: www.gelstat.com

## Imigran Recovery

A treatment designed specifically for migraines that contains sumatriptan and acts on the root cause of the migraine to relieve the four most common symptoms: headache, nausea and sensitivity to light and sound. The tablet form of the medication is available over-the-counter from pharmacies after completing a questionnaire (in pharmacies and on the website) to determine your suitability.

Website: www.imigranrecovery.co.uk

## Kool 'n' Soothe Migraine

Cooling gel sheets that are placed across the forehead to help provide relief from headache. Available from pharmacies and supermarkets nationwide.

Website: www.kobayashihealthcare.co.uk/Kool-N-Soothe

## Lumie

A range of light therapy products, including dawn simulators, light boxes and visors. These products could be helpful if your migraines are linked to Seasonal Affective Disorder or shift work.

Website: www.lumie.com

## McKenzie Lumbar Roll

Recommended for the prevention and treatment of back and neck pain caused by poor posture.

Website: www.backinaction.co.uk

**Midrid**

An over-the-counter preparation for the treatment of migraines and headaches. It contains a combination of paracetamol, for pain relief, and isometheptene mucate, which causes the blood vessels in the brain to narrow. Available over the counter from pharmacies after completing a questionnaire (at high street and online pharmacies) to determine your suitability.

Website: www. expresschemist.co.uk

**Migra-Cap**

A cap designed by a migraineur that provides cold therapy and darkness and has been shown to provide relief for many migraine sufferers.

Website: www.migracap.com

**Migraherb**

A THR herbal medicine containing 100 mg of dried feverfew. Available from pharmacies nationwide.

Website: www.hollandandbarrett.com

**Migraine Buddy**

An app that helps you keep track of your migraines and identify your triggers.

Website: www.migrainebuddy.com

### Migraine Diary

An easy-to-follow diary enabling you to record details of your migraine attacks. The diary lasts for three months and can be started at any time. Available from the Migraine Trust online shop.

Website: diary.migrainetrust.org

### Migraleve

An over-the-counter medication for the treatment of migraine attacks. Migraleve Pink contains paracetamol and codeine to treat the head pain, together with buclizine hydrochloride, an anti-emetic, to relieve the nausea. If taken at the first sign of a migraine, this medication can prevent an attack from developing further. Migraleve Yellow contains paracetamol and codeine and is aimed at treating the continuing migraine symptoms. These must always be taken after the first dose of Migraleve Pink. Migraleve Complete is a pack that contains both the pink and yellow tablets. Available at pharmacies nationwide.

Website: www.migraleve.co.uk

### Migrastick

A roll-on containing mint and lavender essential oils for use on temples, forehead and the nape of the neck to help relieve headache and migraine pain.

Website: www.hollandandbarrett.com

## MigreLief

A range of dietary supplements for the prevention of migraine. The original formula contains 200 mg of riboflavin, 150 mg of magnesium and 50 mg of feverfew whole leaf in each tablet. The recommended dosage is two a day. Other products in the range include one with a fast-acting formula as well as one aimed at children and menstrual migraines.

Website: www.migrelief.com

## The Sea-Band

A knitted, elasticated wristband, which works by applying pressure on the Nei Kuan acupressure point on each wrist by means of a plastic stud. The bands don't use drugs, so they don't cause any of the side effects associated with anti-nausea drugs and can be worn on each wrist whenever you feel nauseous. They are suitable for adults and children and are available in pharmacies across the UK.

Website: www.sea-band.co.uk

# Directory

Below is a list of useful contacts that offer information, advice and support to migraine sufferers.

**British Acupuncture Council**

The British Acupuncture Council (BAcC) is the leading self-regulatory body for the practice of traditional acupuncture in the UK. The website offers factsheets about acupuncture as well as a directory of registered traditional acupuncturists. All BAcC members have undergone degree-level training in traditional acupuncture, Chinese medicine and western biomedical sciences, including anatomy, physiology and pathology, and must comply with the BAcC Code of Safe Practice and Code of Professional Conduct.

Website: www.acupuncture.org.uk

**British Association for the Study of Headache (BASH)**

The United Kingdom national society member of the International Headache Society (IHS) and the European Headache Federation (EHF). Membership is open to all healthcare professionals with an interest in headaches. All members of BASH are automatically made members of the IHS and receive its journal, *Cephalalgia*. The revised second edition BASH Guidelines for the diagnosis and management of migraine and tension-type headache is available to download online.

Website: www.bash.org.uk

**Foods Matter**

Offers information on food allergies and intolerances, including how they may be implicated in some sufferers' migraines.

Website: www.foodsmatter.com

**Headache Expert**

A website set up to offer a reference point on the causes, symptoms and treatments of migraines and headaches. Includes features and articles written by health journalists and experts with a particular interest or background in this area.

Website: www.headacheexpert.co.uk

**Headache UK**

An alliance working for people who suffer from headaches.

Website: www.headacheuk.org

**Help for Headaches**

A US website that offers information and resources intended to help improve the lives of headache and migraine sufferers. The site content is reviewed by a doctor.

Website: www.helpforheadaches.com

**The International Headache Society**

An organisation aimed at professionals working with people whose lives are affected by headache disorders. The website promotes the society and its charitable objectives and activities. It welcomes society members and everyone working or seeking information in the field of headaches. Members receive the society's international journal, *Cephalalgia*.

Website: www.ihs-headache.org

### The International Stress Management Association

A registered charity with a multi-disciplinary professional membership that includes the UK and the Republic of Ireland. It exists to promote sound knowledge and best practice in the prevention and reduction of human stress and provides referrals to stress management professionals. The website offers free factsheets and a stress questionnaire.

Website: www.isma.org.uk

### MAGNUM: Migraine Awareness Group: a National Understanding for Migraineurs

An American non-profit organisation that aims to raise public and government awareness of the medical seriousness of migraines.

Website: www.migraines.org

### Medicines and Healthcare products Regulatory Agency (MHRA)

The government agency responsible for ensuring that medicines and medical devices work and are acceptably safe. Includes a section on the safety of herbal medicines and a full list of herbal medicines granted a traditional herbal registration (THR).

Website: www.mhra.gov.uk

### Migraine.com

A US website that aims to empower patients and caregivers to take control of their migraines by providing a platform to learn, educate and connect with peers and healthcare professionals.

Website: www.migraine.com

## Migraine 4 Kids

A website run by the Migraine Action Association for children and young people with migraines. The site offers easy-to-follow information and advice as well as a new web-based app called MiGain, which enables young people to take better control of their migraines.

Website: www.migraine4kids.org.uk

## Migraine Action

A UK charity that aims to bridge the gap between people affected by migraine and the medical world by providing unbiased information on all aspects of migraine. Also offers a helpline staffed by trained advisers, a specialist headache nurse service and a web forum.

Website: www.migraine.org.uk

## Migraine Association of Ireland

Offers information about migraines, both for sufferers and health professionals. The website has useful downloads, such as a migraine diary sheet and seminar transcripts on a variety of topics. You can subscribe to the charity's free monthly e-zine, *Migra-zine*. Members also receive copies of the newsletter and relevant publications and can access a discussion board.

Website: www.migraine.ie

## Migraine Aura Foundation

A website that explains migraine auras and the classification of visual disturbances. The site includes simulations of migraine auras which are useful to show to non-migraineurs when trying to explain what an aura is like. Also features a Migraine Art section, claiming that migraines have been a major source of inspiration to artists.

Website: www.migraine-aura.com

**The Migraine Trust**

Seeks to empower, inform and support those affected by migraines while providing information for health professionals and actively funding and publicising research. The website includes fact sheets and an online migraine diary you can download for free. The online shop sells a selection of books on migraines.

Website: www.migrainetrust.org

**My Migraine Connection**

Offers information and the latest news on migraines. The clinical content is reviewed by physicians.

Website: www.mymigraineconnection.com

**National Migraine Centre (Formerly known as City of London Migraine Clinic)**

A research centre and outpatient service with more than 30 years of experience in the treatment of headaches and migraines. The clinic's team of registered doctors provides specialist care in a charitable setting. It is a registered charity and social enterprise that is independent of the NHS. Everybody can access the service. You can ask your GP for a referral, or make an appointment directly with the clinic by using the online contact form. The website offers downloadable fact sheets, an online video about coping with migraines and a newsletter containing useful information for migraine sufferers.

Website: www.nationalmigrainecentre.org.uk

**Organisation for the Understanding of Cluster Headaches – OUCH (UK)**

Provides support and information for those who suffer from cluster headaches.

Website: www.ouchuk.org

**Pain Concern**

A website run by chronic pain sufferers. Offers information and support to pain sufferers, their families and carers.

Website: www.painconcern.org.uk

**Relaxation for Living**

Offers courses, DVDs and CDs that aim to teach people how to relax and deal with stress and anxiety, using breathing and muscle relaxation techniques.

Website: www.rfli.co.uk

PERSONAL HEALTH GUIDES

# Anxiety

## A self-help guide to feeling better

Wendy Green

Foreword by Joanne Sale, senior lecturer in mental health, University of Bedfordshire

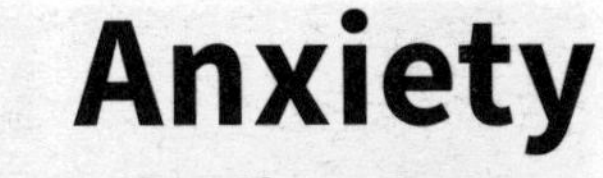


## A self-help guide to feeling better

Wendy Green

£8.99

Paperback

ISBN: 978-1-84953-822-0

In this easy-to-follow book, Wendy Green explains how psychological, genetic and dietary factors can contribute to anxiety and offers practical advice and a holistic approach to help you deal with the symptoms, including simple dietary and lifestyle changes and DIY complementary therapies. Find out 50 things you can do today, including:

- **Replace negative thoughts and behaviour with positive thoughts and behaviour**
- **Manage stress and relax to reduce symptoms**
- **Choose beneficial foods and supplements**
- **Find helpful organisations and products**

PERSONAL HEALTH GUIDES

# IBS

## A self-help guide to feeling better

Wendy Green

Foreword by Dr Nick Read,
chair of The IBS Network